Notes on Gynaecolog

Notes on Gynaecological Nursing

William C. Fream
MB, BS, SRN, BTA Cert. (Hons), STD, FCNA
General Practitioner, Casterton, Victoria, Australia.
Formerly Principal Nurse Educator,
Ballarat Base Hospital, Victoria, Australia

CHURCHILL LIVINGSTONE
EDINBURGH LONDON AND NEW YORK 1979

CHURCHILL LIVINGSTONE
Medical Division of Longman Group Limited

Distributed in the United States of America by
Longman Inc., 19 West 44th Street, New York,
N.Y. 10036, and by associated companies,
branches and representatives throughout
the world.

First published 1979

ISBN 0 443 01480 9

British Library Cataloguing in Publication Data

Fream, William Charles
    Notes on gynaecological nursing.
    1. Gynecologic nursing
    I. Title
    618.1'002'4613   RG105   78-40845

Printed in Singapore by Huntsmen Offset Printing Pte Ltd

Preface

Gynaecology is a highly specialized branch of medicine. The illnesses encountered are of the most intimate variety and many patients have great difficulty in talking about them. Often patients are far more ready to discuss their symptoms, fears and hopes with their nurses than with their doctors and therefore nurses in this field are in a very special position.

This book, like my others in the series, is intended for students preparing themselves for examinations. However, the other books have been found useful by a far wider section of nursing, medical and para-medical personnel than they were written for, and I hope this one is too.

1979   W. C. F.

Contents

Contents

1. Sexual Determination and Development. Intersex

Chromosomal sex

Production of sex cells or gametes involves reduction division. Each gamete contains one half set of chromosomes. Almost all ova contain one X chromosome. (Small proportion have two, XX, chromosomes and an equal proportion contain none. See page 9.) Almost all spermatazoa contain either one X chromosome or one Y chromosome but small proportion contain both, XY, or no sex chromosome.

Combination of ovum and sperm at conception brings together an X chromosome in the ovum and either an X or a Y in the sperm. If two X chromosomes, the individual is female. If X and Y, result is male.

Control of sexual development

The presence of Y chromosome initiates formation of 'organiser substance' which promotes development of male sexual ducts from the Wolffian duct system. Absence of Y chromosomes fails to initiate organiser substance and Wolffian duct system degenerates. Mullerian duct system develops and forms female internal organs. Hence all embryos would tend to female organisation unless presence of Y chromosome dictates formation of organiser substance which alters anatomy to become male.

Sex chromatin

Two X chromosomes occur in all female cells. However, only one needed for efficient functioning of cell. Chromosomal material of redundant X chromosome pushed to side of cell and remains inactive. With suitable staining techniques this chromatin can be revealed. Called Barr bodies. Can be used to prove sex. Fetal cells in amniotic fluid can be obtained before birth to determine sex. Not done as a routine procedure but sex test can be done if amniotic fluid taken for other reasons. Also, there are conditions which can be transmitted to male offspring but not to female and the parents might prefer to abort a pregnancy if it is known that the fetus is male and will suffer the condition. Absence of Barr bodies in fetal cells proves that fetus is male. Such conditions include agammaglobulinaemia, Duchenne muscular dystrophy, amaurotic familial idiocy, choroideraemia, Hunter's syndrome.

In adults technique applied to cells of buccal mucous membrane or to leucocytes to prove chromosomal sex. Used in cases of intersex.

Gonadal sex

Gonads are either ovaries or testicles (testes). Both develop from epithelium separate from tissues which become other internal sexual organs. By 6 weeks gestation gonadal tissue invaded by migrating primordial germ cells from yolk sac. By 7 weeks differentiation into ovary or testis has begun. At 20 weeks ovary contains about 7 million oocytes. About one third of these remain at birth. By 7 years of age about a quarter to half a million remain. During fertile life less than 500 will become mature ova and perhaps only two or three become fertilised.

Testes pass along inguinal canal into scrotum shortly before birth. Occasionally one or both do not descend and if coupled with other anatomical anomalies a mistake as to sex of child can be made. Hence child may be raised as female and present psychological difficulties when error is discovered.

Other causes of apparent female gender occur. (See page 6.)

Sexual organs. Genitalia

In the vast majority of human beings differentiation of sex by appearance of external genitalia is accurate. In a few cases appearances deceptive. Almost always appearance is of female child whereas correct gender is male with anatomical faults. (See page 4.)

Secondary sexual characteristics

Development depends on interplay of hormones — growth, thyroxine, sex — and their pituitary trophic hormones. Final influence results from sensitivity of target organs to androgens; in the male, testosterone mainly, and oestrogens in the female. Androgens bring about enlargement of penis, development of glans, male distribution of body and facial hair, enlargement of larynx with consequent deepening of voice, greater muscle bulk. Oestrogens bring about greater fat bulk, breast development, development of labia, maturation of uterus, female distribution of hair and onset of menstrual flow.

Gender role

All societies have traditional, fairly rigid expectations of male and female behaviour. Children born into societies subjected to subtle pressures from birth onwards by parents, relatives, sibs, teachers, peer groups to behave in ways acceptable to that particular society. Development of secondary sexual characteristics at puberty accentuate and reinforce education for a particular role.

Errors in diagnosing sex at birth occur when external genitalia are ambiguous. Subsequent upbringing imprints for wrong gender role. When true sex eventually determined person may find it too difficult to change from male personality to female or vice versa.

Intersexuality

Any discrepancy between various components of sexual manifestations — chromosomes, genitalia, hormones, gender role — is an intersexual condition.

Classification. Traditionally classified according to type of gonad present: ovarian, testicular, mixed. Ovarian intersex also called female hermophrodism or female pseudohermophrodism. Testicular intersex also called male hermophrodism or male pseudohermophrodism. Mixed intersex also called mixed gonadal dysgenesis, true hermophrodism or ovotesticular intersex.

Ovarian intersex

Definition. Condition in which ovaries present but growth of external genitalia abnormal enough to give rise to uncertainty in determination of sex.

Cause. Presence of androgens in abnormally large amounts. Due to:

1. Oversecretion of androgens by fetal adrenal glands
2. Maternal secretion of androgens due to tumour of adrenal gland
3. Drug induced if mother received one of a number of drugs at critical period of formation of genitalia, between 5th and 10th weeks of gestation

1. Oversecretion of endogenous androgens

Adrenal gland secretes three principle groups of hormones: cortisol, androgens, aldosterone.

Cortisol and androgen production controlled by adrenocorticotrophic hormone (ACTH) from anterior pituitary. Amount of ACTH supressed by circulating cortisol. If cortisol is not produced, or produced in too small quantity, amount of ACTH increased.

In major form of ovarian intersex defect in production of cortisol occurs due to deficiency in an enzyme (C21 hydroxylase) in adrenal gland. Hence too much ACTH produced by pituitary. Enzyme defect does not affect androgen production and under influence of excessive ACTH large amounts of androgen circulate. This caused developmental anomalies of external genitalia in female fetuses and precocious puberty (early maturation of sexual functioning) in males.

If enzyme deficiency severe aldosterone as well as cortisol is absent. Hence sodium chloride is lost in urine and severe electrolyte imbalance occurs rapidly and may cause death if not diagnosed early.

Other enzymes which play parts in production of adrenal hormones may be deficient (but far less commonly than C21-hydroxylase). These are C11 hydroxylase, C17-hydroxylase, 3-betahydroxysteroid dehydrogenase. In addition to intersex difficulties other effects may be present, e.g. hypertension.

2. Maternal androgens

When present during pregnancy ovarian intersex may arise. However, at birth, maternal androgen stimulus removed and genital anomalies progress no further.

3. Exogenous maternal drugs

Several drugs implicated: testosterone, progesterone,

diethylstilboestrol. Most common is progesterone used to prevent abortion where this has threated in first trimester.

Presentation. External genitalia. Range from normal with nothing more than a large clitoris to very large clitoris mistaken for penis, with a combined urethral/vaginal (urogenital sinus) opening at base of clitoris mistaken for hypospadiac urethra, and fusion of labia. Scrotal skin never occurs and ovaries never descend out of pelvis. Internal organs always normal.

Electrolyte imbalance may cause vomiting, wasting, dehydration and circulatory collapse.

Diagnosis. Careful examination of external genitalia essential in all cases where testes and scrotum absent.

Differentiation between small penis and abnormal clitoris not always easy.

All urine saved and 24 hour specimens tested for:

Urinary 17 ketosteroids

Pregnanetriol

Blood collected for sodium chloride and potassium levels. Serum cortisol level determined.

Exploration of urogenital sinus under general anaesthetic, possibly with X-rays after injection of radio-opaque dye.

Later, if further proof required, chromosome studies will show Barr bodies in at least 25 per cent of buccal cells.

Treatment. Correction of electrolyte imbalance may be life saving initially. ACTH supression achieved by administration of cortisone. Infant dose 25 mg/day. As child grows dose increased up to 100 mg/day according to urinary 17 ketosteroid and pregnanetriol excretion. Lower doses of prednisone may be used instead, 2·5 mg b.d. for infants, increasing to 10 mg b.d.

Surgery to external genitalia performed at 3 to 4 years of age. Child is female and fully normal and functional internally. Clitorisectomy and widening of introitus may be sufficient. Vaginoplasty may be required later.

Testicular intersex

Definition. Condition in which testes present but internal and/or external genitalia abnormal enough to be ambiguous. Patients always sterile.

Types
1. Abnormal external genitalia who develop male secondary sexual characteristics at puberty.
2. Female external genitalia who develop female secondary sexual characteristics at puberty. (Androgen insensitivity syndrome).
3. Ambiguous external genitalia. Absent internal genitalia except for non-maturing testes. Female secondary sexual characteristics at puberty, but menstruation does not occur.

Type 1
May have normal external genitalia except for undescended testes. Commonly small penis with hypospadias. Wrinkled scrotal skin present but empty. May resemble labia majora. Frequently inguinal hernia. During repair of hernia presence of fallopian tubes and uterus discovered.

At puberty, penis grows, voice deepens, facial and body hair develops.

Diagnosis. Often condition unsuspected and undiagnosed until examined for insurance, or prior to induction into forces or when patient requests examination before marriage.

Buccal smear shows normal XY chromosome pattern with no Barr bodies.

Occasionally child raised as female. Absence of menstruation leads to investigation.

Treatment. If child raised as female and has well developed feminine gender role, surgical conversion to more female anatomy advised — clitorisectomy, vaginoplasty, orchidectomy, mammoplasty or stimulation of breast development with oestrogen therapy.

Type 2
(Androgen insensitivity syndrome)
External genitalia usually markedly female and good breast development at puberty. Pubic hair usually absent or scanty. Failure to menstruate usual complaint bringing patient for investigation.

Diagnosis. Absent fallopian tubes and uterus. Blind vagina which may be short. Buccal smear shows absent Barr bodies. Chromosome studies show male 46:XY karyotype. Plasma testosterone levels normal male level. Oestrogen levels usually higher than normal male levels but lower than normal female.

Treatment. Physical treatment usually unnecessary. Psychological understanding and careful considerate support essential. Patient regards herself as female in every way apart from failure to menstruate. She is sterile however. This information should be imparted with empathy and ample opportunity given to discuss all its implications.

Orchidectomy sometimes advised because of increased risk of malignant change. When performed ethinyl oestradiol 0·02 mg daily for 21 days each month prescribed to prevent development of menopausal signs and symptoms.

Type 3

Apparently female external genitalia but with 'clitoris' large enough to assign male gender at birth. Child raised as boy but develops breasts at puberty.

Diagnosis. Careful examination. Buccal smear shows no Barr bodies. Chromosome studies show normal male 46:XY karyotype. Urine shows high 17 ketosteroids and pregnanetriol. Laparotomy to detect testes and absence of fallopian tubes and uterus.

Treatment. Depends largely on gender role. If raised as girl clitoridectomy and vaginoplasty. If raised as boy, urethroplasty and closure of hypospadias. Mastectomy.

Generally speaking conversion to female surgically easier than vice versa.

Mixed (ovotesticular) intersex (very rare)

Definition. Gonads contain both testicular and ovarian elements. Patient displays aspects of both male and female anatomy and histology.

Presentation. Ambiguous external genitalia, often with one testis in inguinal canal or scrotum. Commonly breast development at puberty and onset of menstruation in person brought up as male. More common in Negroes.

Diagnosis. Biopsy of suspected gonads shows either testis on one side with ovary on other or one gonad containing both types of tissue. Internal genitalia show fallopian tube associated with ovary and vas deferens associated with testis.

Y chromosome seen in about half. Barr bodies present in buccal smear but in smaller proportion of cells than in females.

Treatment. Depends on gender role. Every effort made to eradicate female organs when child raised as boy and male organs when child raised as girl.

When one whole gonad is ovary, person has good chance of normal fertile female development. Testis rarely functions normally and male always sterile.

2. Chromosomal Abnormalities

Meiosis ensures equal division of 46 chromosomes into two equal lots of 23 in daughter cells. Twenty-two of these are autosomal chromosomes and one sex chromosome. Ova contain one X sex chromosome. Spermatozoa contain either one X or one Y chromosome. At fertilisation ovarian X chromosome meets sperm X chromosome to produce female child with 44 XX karyotype or ovarian X chromosome meets sperm Y chromosome to produce male child with 44:XY karyotype.

Occasionally meiosis goes wrong and ova produced with two X chromosomes (22:XX), or with no X chromosome (22:0) and spermatazoa produced with both X and Y (22:XY) or with none (22:0).

When conception occurs between such gametes abnormal development can occur.

Possibilities:

Ovum		Sperm			
22:XX	+	22:XY	=	44:XXXY	Abnormal male
22:XX	+	22:0	=	44:XX	Normal female
22:0	+	22:XY	=	44:XY	Normal male
22:0	+	22:0	=	44.00	Lethal

When an abnormal gamete fuses with a normal one the possibilities are:

Ovum		Sperm			
22:X	+	22:XY	=	44:XXY	Abnormal male Kleinfelter's syndrome
22:XX	+	22:X	=	44:XXX	Infertile female 'Pure' gonadal dysgenesis
22:XX	+	22:Y	=	44:XXY	Abnormal male Kleinfelter's syndrome
22:0	+	22:X	=	44:X0	Abnormal female Turner's syndrome
22:0	+	22:0	=	44:00	Lethal
22:X	+	22:0	=	44:X0	Abnormal female Turner's syndrome

Only two of these possibilities are of gynaecological interest here. Turner's syndrome and 'pure' gonadal dysgenesis.

Turner's syndrome (gonadal dysgenesis)

Definition. Condition in which apparently normal female fails to develop secondary sexual characteristics.

Signs and symptoms. Typical body form — short stature (less than 150 cm), webbed neck, wide carrying angle at elbows, shield chest with wide space between nipples, occasionally coarctation of aorta.

Primary amenorrhoea and failure of breast development often presenting symptoms.

Diagnosis. Examination reveals infantile genitalia and breasts. Chromosomal studies show 44:X0 pattern. Buccal smear shows absent Barr bodies. Hormone studies show childhood levels of oestrogen and raised level of follicle stimulating hormone (FSH). If laparotomy performed for other reasons, rudimentary gonads observed.

Treatment. To stimulate breast development and avoid premature menopause, ethinyl oestradiol 0·05 to 0·15 mg given 3 weeks per month. When given as combination contraceptive pill, proliferative build up of endometrium prevented by presence of progestogen. Patient remains sterile but is otherwise healthy female.

Pure gonadal dysgenesis

Definition. Condition in which there is total absence of gonadal tissue.

Presentation. Usually girl with primary amenorrhoea absent breast development and no pubic hair growth. Normal height.

Diagnosis. Buccal smear not helpful. May or may not show Barr bodies. Chromosome studies may show normal female 46:XX, normal male 46:XY or mosaic mixtures, e.g. 45:XO/46:XX. Necessary to distinguish between gonadal dysgenesis and pituitary failure when 46:XX pattern shown. Hormones in former are absent or low oestrogen, high FSH and LH. In latter FSH, LH and oestrogen all low. Further proof of pituitary insufficiency if urinary oestrogens rise follow administration of FSH.

Treatment. Replacement hormones. Ethinyl oestradiol 0·02 mg daily for 3 weeks each month. Girl will be sterile but acceptable breast growth and avoidance of menopausal symptoms.

3. Female Sex Hormones

Hypothalamus, pituitary, ovaries and placenta involved in hormone production.

Hypothalamus

No nerve connections between anterior pituitary and brain. Rich vascular connection between hypothalamus and anterior pituitary. Hypothalamus produces releasing hormones (RH) one of which causes release of follicle stimulating hormone (FSH) and luteinising hormone (LH).

RH production influenced by nerve connections between hypothalamus and other parts of brain hence emotional and stress factors play part in ultimate sex hormone release. Normally FSH-RH produced cyclically in females and carried to anterior pituitary. Also influenced by circulating oestrogens.

Anterior pituitary

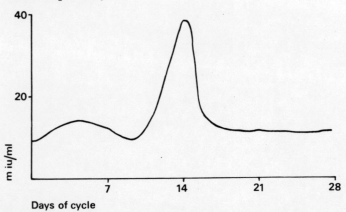

Fig. 1 Plasma FSH

Two gonadotrophins produced, FSH and LH. Former produced in very low concentration until puberty (less than 10 i.u./day urinary). Slight increase then until onset of menstruation. Thereafter, cyclic production (between 10 and 70 i.u./day) rising in first half of menstrual cycle and peaking at ovulation. At menopause cyclic production ceases and reaches high constant levels.

LH production practically immeasurable at menstruation. Rises suddenly to high peak just before ovulation, falls immediately to low level then rises slightly during second half of menstrual cycle.

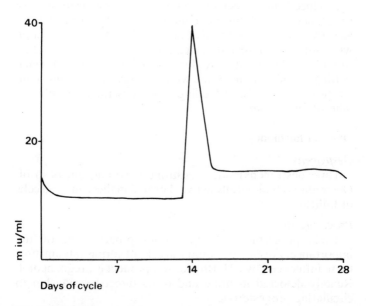

Fig. 2 Plasma LH

Function of FSH and LH

FSH stimulates development of follicles in ovary. Granulosa cells produce more oestrogen and ovum matures. When lacking, follicles fail to mature; possible cause of infertility (q.v.).

LH enhances development and maturity of corpus luteum after ovulation. LH will not function unless FSH also present.

Prolactin

Prolactin also produced by anterior pituitary. Normally supressed by an inhibitory factor produced in hypothalamus in response to circulating oestrogen and progesterone. When oestrogen and progesterone fall to low level immediately after childbirth, prolactin production increases and milk production starts.

Oxytocin

Produced in detectable amounts in last trimester of pregnancy. Causes uterine contractions at full term. Uterus sensitive to oxytocin at this time. Production also increased when nipples stimulated during suckling. Causes contraction of milk glands and storage ducts so that milk flows. Termed 'letting down' of milk. Some women experience uterine contractions during breast feeding which described by some as 'almost an orgasm'.

Ovarian hormones

Oestrogens

Three oestrogens made — oestrone, oestradiol and oestriol. Oestradiol is biologically active. Formed in theca interna cells of follicles.

Progestagens

Three progestagens formed. Only progesterone of any importance. Formed by granulosa cells of corpus luteum after these influenced by LH. Breakdown product is pregnanediol. Readily detected in urine and bears direct relationship to circulating progesterone.

Patterns of production

Oestrogens. Up to 10 years oestrogen production low. Thereafter doubles until onset of menstruation. Throughout fertile years production is cyclical gradually increasing from end of menstruation to mid-cycle reaching peak just before ovulation.

Immediate fall at ovulation and second more sustained peak in second half of cycle with fall to very low level before onset of menstruation.

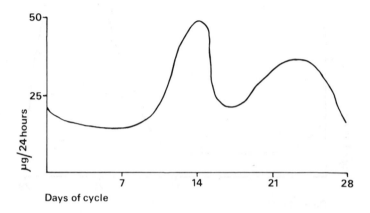

Fig. 3 Urinary oestrogens

During pregnancy oestrogen level increases to 400 times non-pregnancy level. Increase is gradual throughout pregnancy reaching maximum at full term. Falls abruptly immediately after delivery. Source of maternal oestrogen is placenta. Urinary oestradiol levels during pregnancy good source of information regarding placental efficiency.

High level of oestrogen during last weeks of pregnancy may affect newborn causing gynaecomastia and vaginal bloody discharge.

Progesterone. Production almost undetectable until puberty. Rises to peak 7 days after ovulation. Falls to former low level before menstruation.

After menopause progesterone level falls to almost undetectable levels. Probably adrenal glands source of this.

During pregnancy placenta takes over progesterone production. Gradual increase to 24 weeks then rapidly to plateau at 34 weeks and sudden fall after delivery to undetectable level.

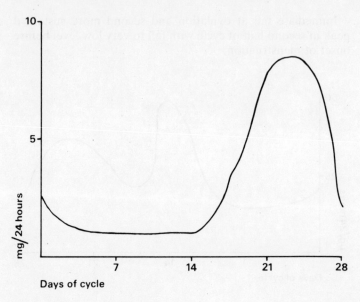

Fig. 4 Urinary pregnanediol

Effects of oestrogens and progesterone
Oestrogens
1. Maturation of uterus, vagina, external genitalia
2. Development of secondary sexual characteristics, increased fat deposition with female distribution, growth of breasts, growth of pubic and axillary hair, fine skin texture
3. Development of endometrium cyclically each month (Proliferative phase)
4. Suppression of FSH and FSH-RH by negative feedback.
During pregnancy enhances placental formation and maintenance, relaxes cervix at term, growth and mobility of nipples, relaxes ligaments generally.
Progesterone
1. Development of endometrium cyclically each month (Secretory phase)
2. Alters cervical mucus making it tenacious and impenetrable

3. Prepares endometrium for implantation
4. Early development of placenta
5. Aids in development of glands, for lactation
6. Inhibits myometrial excitability during pregnancy.

Other female hormones

Human chorionic gonadotrophin (HCG)

Produced by trophoblast during pregnancy. Reaches peak about 60 to 80 days after implantation. Falls to low but detectable level during rest of pregnancy. Disappears within 48 hours of delivery.

Functions. Little precise known. Causes maintenance of corpus luteum during first trimester. Possibly causes development of Leydig cells in male fetal testes, and hence essential for production of male organiser substance which brings about male differentiation.

HCG excreted in urine and is basis for modern pregnancy tests.

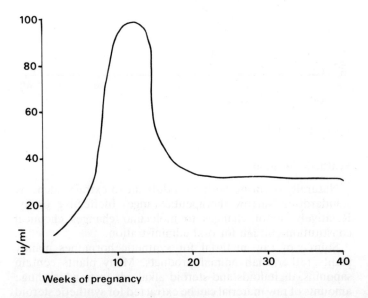

Fig. 5 Serum HCG

Human placental lactogen (HPL)

Produced by trophoblast during pregnancy. Appears early and rises to maximum by term. Little known of its functions. Resembles growth hormone but almost none passes to fetus. Possible increases placental transfer of nutrients. Influences breast preparation for lactation.

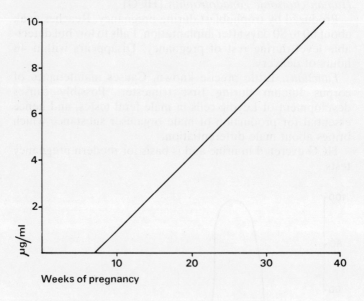

Fig. 6 Serum HPL

Synthetic hormones

Naturally occuring hormones difficult to extract, identify, standardise. Narrow therapeutic range. Ineffective orally. Relatively minor changes to molecular changes chemical constitution enough for oral administration.

Source of raw material for synthetic hormones mainly plants rather than animal products. Many plants contain saponins, digitaloids and steroid alkaloids from which huge amounts of raw material can be extracted for synthetic steroid production.

Stilbene group

Stilboestrol manufactured very early. Used for many years to supress lactation, to prevent early abortion, in male carcinoma prostate. Rarely used now. Implicated in early carcinoma of vagina in young females when mother given drug in early pregnancy.

Dienoestrol is weakly oestrogenic. Useful as topical application in senile vaginitis.

Oestradiol group

Ethinyl oestradiol is 20 times more powerful than naturally occuring oestrogens. Most common synthetic oestrogen. Used extensively in contraceptive pill, for control of hypermenorrhoea and dysmenorrhoea, supression of lactation, postmenopausal syndromes. Effective orally.

Mestranol is similar to ethinyl oestradiol and is an alternative form of oestrogen used in contraceptive pill.

Oestradiol valerate is weak oestrogen. Much used in postmenopausal syndromes.

Chlorotrianisene group

One useful derivative is clomiphene citrate. Antioestrogen. Suppresses effects of oestrogen and encourages production of FSH-RF and FSH itself. Formerly used as 'fertility pill' in female infertility.

Other sources of hormones

Urine of pregnant mares. Rich source of equine oestrogen. Marketed as Premarin. Weakly oestrogenic in humans. Not nauseating. Used primarily for post-menopausal syndromes.

Human menopausal urine

Contains human gonadotrophins. Useful to initiate ovulation and in female infertility.

4. Menstrual Cycle. Disorders of Menstruation

At puberty hypothalamus matures and cyclical production of FSH-RF increases. Age of maturation from 8 to 18 years, commonly about 11 or 12. In response to RF, FSH released from anterior pituitary. Influences ovaries to ripen follicles. Theca interna cells produce oestrogens which carried in blood stream to all organs. Effect on endometrium particularly.

Endometrium undergoes proliferative phase for approximate 7 to 10 days from end of last menstrual flow. Ovulation occurs because of sudden spurt of FSH and LH. Discharged follicle organised into corpus luteum and produces progesterone.

Progesterone causes endometrium to continue to develop for next 14 days — secretory phase — so called because of storage of glycogen and other nutrient granules in epithelial cells.

Oestrogen also causes negative feedback to hypothalamus and pituitary reducing RH and FSH. Without their influence ovarian production ceases and circulating oestrogen and progesterone falls away. Endometrial cells cannot sustain themselves with too little hormone and shed as menstrual flow.

Cycle usually repeats about every 28 days but few women are utterly regular. Flow lasts 2 to 6 days but again variation from woman to woman and from month to month. Notation used to denote length of period and of cycle is fraction, thus 3/28 denotes 3 day duration in a 28 day cycle.

Endometrial changes

End of flow. Tips of glands remaining. Lining of cuboidal or low columnar cells proliferate and extend over raw surface.

Day 6 to 14. Great increase in blood vessels, and stroma cells. Gland pits become long and tortuous.

Day 14. Vacuoles deep to epithelial nuclei.

Day 16 to 28. Vast increase in vacuoles. Gradual migration of vacuoles from depth of cell to surface superficial to nuclei.

Day 28. Blood vessels withdraw from surface.

Bleeding occurs between deepest (spongy) layer of endometrium and overlying layers. Sloughing and liquification of overlying layers.

Menses. 50 to 150 ml containing 25 to 75 mg iron, cell debris, mucus, sodium, potassium, chloride, phosphate. Does not clot unless in excessive amounts.

Other changes during cycle

Cervix retains its epithelium. Cervical glands produce copious watery mucus under influence of oestrogen. Mucus becomes thicker and tenacious under influence of progesterone. Specimen of mucus spread on slide assumes frosted fern-like pattern as it dries when under oestrogen influence. Most marked at time of ovulation. When progesterone present mucus much more tenacious. Can be drawn out to threadlike form. Ferning and thread formation (spinbarkeit) used as crude test of ovulation.

Vaginal cells not shed at menstruation but undergo changes during cycle. Vagina covered with wet surface squamous epithelium. During proliferative phase, shed surface cells are flat and separate with few leucocytes. During secretory phase cells tend to clump, have curled up edges and many leucocytes present.

Proportion of each type of cell can be used to indicate stage of cycle and whether ovulation has occured. (No ovulation, no progesterone ∴ no secretory phase cells.)

Myometrial effects. Uterus tends to contract rhythmically and imperceptibly under influence of oestrogen. More forcibly and more sustained under progesterone. Progesterone thought to be cause of menstrual pain in early cycles.

General effects. Salt and water retained under influence of progesterone. More marked in some women. Every cell in body retains fluid. May be cause of irritability, mild headaches and tension pre-menstrually.

Breast fullness and tenderness frequent. Possibly due to water retention but more likely direct oestrogen effect.

Temperature rises by 0·5 to 1° C. at ovulation. Progesterone has thermogenic effect. Basis for 'ovulation' or 'cyclic' method of contraception (q.v.).

Oestrogen has some effect on calcium metabolism. At menopause less calcium laid down and bones may become osteoporotic.

Disorders of menstruation

Definitions

Amenorrhoea. Absent periods.

Oligomenorrhoea. Cycle extends to 2 weeks or more longer than it used to.

Cryptomenorrhoea. Concealed or retained menses.

Menorrhagia or hypermenorrhoea. Heavy periods but normal length cycle, e.g. 7/28.

Polymenorrhoea or epimenorrhoea. More frequent and heavier periods, e.g. 7/21.

Metrorrhagia. Completely irregular in time, duration frequency and amount.

Intermenstrual bleeding. Some slight loss occurs between periods but does not amount to a period.

Amenorrhoea

Absence of menstruation. Normal before puberty, during pregnancy and lactation, and after menopause. Not a disease in itself. Always a symptom.

Primary amenorrhoea. Never started menstruating.

Secondary amenorrhoea. Has had at least one normal period.

Primary amenorrhoea

Normal menstrual pattern usually established by 16 years.
Causes
1. General systemic illnesses. Malnutrition. Tuberculosis. Renal disease. Anaemia. In tropical countries malaria, hookworm infestation
2. Endocrine disorders
   a. Pituitary dwarfism (Lorraine type). Dystrophia adiposogenitalis (Fröhlich's syndrome)
   b. Ovarian. Gonadal dysgenesis (see page 10). Bilateral polycystic ovary (see page 91)

   c. Testes. Testicular intersex (see page 5)
   d. Adrenals. Adreno-genital syndrome (see page 4)
   e. Thyroid. Cretinism
3. Chromosomal abnormalities — Turner's syndrome (see page 10).

Secondary amenorrhoea
   Patient has menstruated normally in past.
   Causes
1. General systemic disorders. Almost any illness can cause temporary amenorrhoea. Of no consequence. Menstruation resumes with recovery from illness. More prolonged effect from tuberculosis, chronic nephritis
2. Psychological. Higher brain centres affect hypothalamus and can supress releasing factors, e.g. anxiety for any reason, guilt feelings, grief reactions, obesity, anorexia nervosa
3. Endocrine disorders
   a. Pituitary. Tumours. Basophil adenoma interferes with FSH and LH production. Chromophobe adenoma, craniopharyngioma, any other space occupying lesion within cranium may cause pressure symptoms on pituitary. Galactorrhoea (Chiari-Frommel syndrome). Persistence of lactation with suppression of FSH and LH
     Trauma. Fractures through base of skull involving middle fossa may damage pituitary portal system. Hence RF's unable to reach anterior pituitary with no secretion of FSH and LH
     Post-partum pituitary necrosis (Sheehan's syndrome) Thrombosis of pituitary portal vessels following massive post-partum haemorrhage
   b. Ovarian. Destruction from surgery or irradiation. Cystic conditions with high oestrogen output. Tumours with high oestrogen output — granulosa cell tumour. Stein-Leventhal syndrome in which ovary becomes cystic with thickened tough surface (see page 91). Arrhenoblastoma coupled with masculinisation (see page 90)
   c. Adrenals. Cushing's disease of adrenal origin. Hyperplasia causes oversecretion of androgens with masculin-

isation and involution of uterus, growth of clitoris, growth of body and facial hair

4. Local causes. Destruction of endometrium by infection, puerperal, tuberculous, irradiation, Asherman's syndrome due to too vigorous or too frequent curettage. Hysterectomy.

Investigations. Careful and detailed history essential. Almost always, diagnosis can be made on this alone.

General examination to include appearance, height, weight, blood pressure, distribution of hair, texture of skin, distribution of fat, state of breast development, palpation of kidneys.

Vaginal examination, inspection of labia, clitoris, perineum. Palpation of inguinal regions. Passage of speculum to visualise cervix, vaginal walls. Passage of sound to determine uterine size. Bimanual examination of uterus and adnexae for size, mobility, tumours or other masses.

Further investigations depend on suspected cause:

1. Histology. Vaginal cytology and endometrial biopsy for ovarian hormone assessment
2. Urinary oestrogens, pregnanediol and 17 oxy- and hydroxysteroids levels
3. Gonadotrophin stimulation test to distinguish between pituitary and ovarian failure. Human menopausal gonadotrophin 100 i.u. injected on alternate days × 3. 24 hour urine collected 7th day for oestrone estimation. If less than 5 μg ovaries have failed to respond. If over 100 μg ovaries normal and pituitary failed
4. Buccal smear and chromosome studies for vaginal atresia, absent uterus or ambiguous genitalia
5. Culdoscopy or laparoscopy to visualise internal genitalia in hypogonadism
6. Radiology-Skull for pituitary fossa when pituitary tumour suspected. IVP may reveal adrenal tumour. Gynaegram may show enlarged ovaries: hysterogram in Asherman's syndrome
7. Laparotomy. To see state of internal organs.

Treatment. Treat the cause if possible.

Psychogenic — sympathetic ear. Supportive counselling. Removal of cause of fear, guilt. Reassurance that amenorrhoea not harmful and will correct itself.

Many of causes of primary amenorrhoea not amenable to correction and patient is sterile. Others such as infections, chronic debilitating disease, need treatment and amenorrhoea will correct itself.

If patient does not wish to become pregnant no need to institute therapy to bring about ovulation. Amenorrhoea, of itself, not an illness. Many patients will accept situation if given adequate explanation and reassurance. Some prefer regular periods even when they know they are not true menstruation but are withdrawal bleeds. These can have combination oestrogen/progestogen contraceptive pill.

If patient wants children stimulation of ovary required. (See 'Infertility', page 27.)

Menorrhagia
Definition. Excessive bleeding either from prolonged periods (menstaxis) or heavy period for normal duration.

Causes. Concomitant infections. Blood dyscrasias. Anticoagulant therapy. Vitamin C deficiency. Anovulatory cycles with no progesterone secretion to oppose continued proliferation.

Local inflammation — salpingitis, pelvic cellulitis. Local tumours, polyps, fibroids, adenomyosis.

Diagnosis. Careful history. General examination. Vaginal examination for state of uterus and adnexae.

Laboratory investigation to exclude blood dyscrasias and determine anaemia. White cell count and sedimentation rate to discover bacterial infections. Hormone levels.

Examination under anaesthesia followed by dilatation and curettage. Scrapings examined for state of endometrium — secretory, proliferative, atrophic, presence of abnormal cells.

Treatment. In dysfunctional bleeding (that in which no cause is discovered), hormones given. Norethisterone 20 to 30 mg orally for 4 days, or 17 hydroxprogesterone caproate 125 to 250 mg single intramuscular injection. Withdrawal bleed like normal period follows in 3 to 5 days. Alternatively norethisterone continued for 20 days and then withdrawn.

Ordinary combination oestrogen/progestogen contraceptive pill controls menstruation very well. Provides stimulus to endometrium to progress to adequate maturity and regression on stopping pill so that bleeding takes place. Can be used for 3 to 6 cycles and then stopped for endogenous control to resume.

Where scrapings show cystic hyperplasia (Swiss cheese pattern of varying sizes of glandular and cyst-like spaces), there is absence of progesterone. Endometrium stimulated to progress to luteal phase with norethisterone 5 mg daily from day 20 to 25 or dydrogesterone 5 mg. Where menorrhogia has functional basis this is corrected.

Hysterectomy may be necessary over 40 years of age when it is quite certain that the menorrhagia is not a conversion symptom of underlying psychological disturbance.

Menstruation in puberty

Menstruation may be quite regular in frequency and duration from start. Often irregular.

Frequently, early periods are anovulatory. Without ovulation corpus luteum not formed, hence progesterone not secreted and endometrium does not progress to secretory phase. If endometrium remains in proliferative phase breakdown only partial and patchy or does not occur at all. Eventually thick bulky endometrium and thickened myometrium. Period then prolonged and/or copious.

Treatment. Reassurance that irregularity not unusual at first. Usually self limiting. Oestrogens avoided as their mode of action is to suppress gonadotrophins and hence they prevent establishment of normal pattern at this age. Norethisterone 5 mg b.d. by injection from day 15 to 25. This converts endometrium from proliferative to secretory phase and withdrawal bleed occurs on ceasing injections. May be repeated over three cycles and next few cycles observed for normal pattern.

Cryptomenorrhoea

Definition. Menstrual flow retained.

Causes. Imperforate hymen. Absent vagina. Rarely cervical stenosis after cone biopsy.

Signs and symptoms. No menstrual flow at puberty. Periodic pains. Menses collect in vagina. Serum reabsorbed and remaining material becomes thick. May persist for months or years causing surprisingly little discomfort. Blood may distend uterus and tubes. Hymen bulges. Looks blue because of blood behind. Occasionally, frequency, retention of urine. Pain in perineum worse while sitting.

Examination. Mass rising out of pelvis. Vagina distended on P.R. examination. Bulging blue hymen.

Treatment. Cruciate incision through hymen. Manual expression to evacuate pent up menses. Careful perineal hygiene to prevent infection. Antibiotic cover for a month. Tetracycline 250 mg q.i.d.

Precocious puberty

Definition. Onset of menses before 10 years.

Causes. Early normal maturation. Pituitary tumour. Encephalitis. Meningitis.

Treatment. Exclude pituitary tumour. Skull X-ray to visualise pituitary fossa. Hormone studies. Test visual fields for optic nerve pressure.

Dysmenorrhoea

Definition. Painful menstruation. Many women suffer discomfort before or during period. Term, dysmenorrhoea applied when severe enough to require treatment.

Types. Primary — present from menarche. Secondary — after years of painless menstruation.

Primary dysmenorrhoea

Causes. Many theories. No proofs.
1. Obstruction to free flow of menses; narrow os, acutely anteverted uterus, retroverted uterus
2. Psychological. Maternal or sibling 'priming' with warnings of their dreadful experiences especially if the person is highly strung
3. Sedentary type of life. Not so common among physically active women
4. Hormonal. Imbalance between oestrogen and progesterone. Predominance of oestrogen causing uterine contraction
5. Prostaglandins. Prostaglandin-$F2\alpha$ released causing contraction of smooth muscle
6. Myometrial 'colic'. Sudden bleeding within uterus causes mechanical pressure which stimulates forcible contraction. 'Mini labour pains.'

Pattern. Usually severe immediately prior to menstrual flow and ceases within 12 hours of start. Pain described as cramping, intermittent or colicky, centred in low abdomen radiating to iliac fossae or thighs.

May be very severe causing shock like symptoms, pallor, coldness, sweating, rapid shallow respirations, weakness. May be accompanied by headache, nausea, vomiting.

Treatment. Reassurance. Enlightenment where this is lacking. Information regarding normality of menstruation. Simple analgesics, paracetamol progressing to paracetamol plus codeine, to dextropropoxyphene or papaverine with atropine and paracetamol, to pentazocine.

In very severe cases pethedine and anti-emetic such as Stemetil used. Best avoided so as not to establish psychological dependence each month.

Supression of ovulation with combination contraceptive pill most common treatment. Almost any pill suitable but preference given to low oestrogen ones. Some firms market pill by alternative name and without enclosed literature regarding contraception.

Dilation of cervix used to be commonly practised but effectiveness only about 20 per cent and incidence of incompetent os reputed to be higher when performed.

Condition self limiting and cured by pregnancy.

Secondary dysmenorrhoea

Causes. Uterine. Endometriosis (see page 70). Fibromata (see page 71). Polyps. Fixed retroversion (see page 68). Extra-uterine pelvic inflammation from any cause.

Signs and symptoms. Pain commencing *after* bleeding starts. Progresses to severe during menstruation. Eases as menstruation ends. Not easily localised.

Treatment. Careful examination to determine associated abnormality. Correction of this where possible.

Occasionally, where pain intractable, presacral neurectomy performed. Hysterectomy may be requested when no further family required.

5. Infertility

Definition
Inability to conceive though apparently normal.

Causes
Male — lack of sufficient viable spermatazoa due to deficiency of FSH or interstitial cell stimulating hormone (ICSH), aspermia, failure of sperms to develop normally, occlusion of vasa deferentia through previous infection.

When sperms are normal — impotence, ignorance, premature ejaculation.

Female — tubal obstruction, excessive acidity of vagina, anovulatory cycles, immunological destruction of sperm, endometrial deficiency, presence of fibroma, carcinoma, polyp.

Investigations
Detailed questioning of both partners may reveal faulty sex techniques, ignorance, impotence. Relative aspermia may result from too frequent intercourse.

Seminal analysis. Semen collected into condom during intercourse, condom free from spermicidal lubricant, or by masturbation. Normal analysis shows up to 5 ml volume with 50 to 150 million sperms/ml, 80 per cent fully motile and less than 25 per cent abnormal forms. Sterility if less than 20 million/ml, more than 20 per cent immotile or more than 40 per cent abnormal.

Testicular biopsy may reveal pathology of testes.

Huhner's test performed for destruction of sperm. Sperm collected from vagina by aspiration immediately after intercourse. Less than 75 per cent motile indicates immunological destruction or too acid medium.

Examination of cervical mucus. After ovulation character of cervical mucus alters. Until progesterone production reaches

high enough levels mucus remains watery and easily pene-
trated by sperms. Under influence of progesterone, mucus
becomes thick and impenetrable.

Ovulation tests. At ovulation corpus luteum develops.
Progesterone level rises. Changes brought about by progesterone taken as evidence that ovulation has occured, e.g.
endometrium shows secretory pattern, vaginal wall desquam-
ates small, round, granular cells which clump together, basal
body temperature rises $0.5°$ C, ferning or cervical mucus fails
to occur.

Direct measurement of oestrogen, progesterone, FSH, LH
now performed by immunoassay on blood or urine.

Tests of tubal patency. Rubins test. Carbon dioxide blown
through tube fitting tightly into cervix. Manometer shows
pressure of gas within uterus and fallopian tubes. At 200 mm
Hg pressure stethoscope placed over left and right iliac fossae
may detect hiss of escaping gas through fimbriae of each tube.
If pressure stays at 200 mm Hg when gas turned off both tubes
are blocked. If pressure falls off rapidly at least one tube is
patent.

Hysterosalpingography more informative than Rubins'
test. Introduction of radio-opaque material shows whether
tubes are patent and reveals abnormalities of uterus if shape of
cavity altered.

Curettings of endometrium reveal presence of cancer cells,
tuberculosis, fibroma or fibrosis.

Treatment

Depends on revealed causative factors if any. Often no
abnormality detected. Advice then needed to ensure highest
chance of conception — reduction of frequency of coitus to
ensure high sperm counts; intercourse soon after ovulation
detected by careful temperature recording; following intercourse, dorsal position maintained for 2 hours with buttocks
or foot of bed raised to facilitate sperm retention.

Anovulation may have pituitary or ovarian causes. Correction not always possible, but replacement of pituitary hormones may stimulate ovaries. Human pituitary gonadotrophin injected on alternate days for 14 days. Human
chorionic gonadotrophin on 12th day acts like LH and ovulation usually occurs.

Clomiphene antagonises effect of circulating oestrogen and secretion of FSH increases. Fifty mg orally for 5 days is followed by ovulation after further 5 days. Clomiphene also used to stimulate male spermatogenesis, 100 mg on alternate days for 4 months.

Tubal obstruction sometimes overcome by incision through obstruction and sewing edges open — salpingostomy — or excision of blocked section and end-to-end anastomosis using operating microscope. Ovaries inspected at same time, adhesions freed, tumours removed. Excision of cornual obstruction and re-implantation of tubes or implantation of ovary into wall of uterus sometimes tried.

6. Sexuality

Few human activities surrounded by so much ignorance, intolerance, prejudice as sexuality. Throughout nature copulation occurs for procreation. Only humans copulate for its own intrinsic pleasure. In some societies this fact accepted and subject is not one to be either paraded or hidden from discussion. Western society has double standards only slowly dissolving. Male may satisfy sexual urge with any consenting partner. Female must remain celibate until she marries when she becomes exclusive property of one man. If a woman steps outside the boundaries laid down by society she is still considered by many to be of lesser worth and not acceptable.

Gradual enlightenment, and growing demand to throw off false standards, has done much to remove the hold on peoples' behaviour exercised for so long by self appointed arbiters of right and wrong.

Psychologists such as Freud lifted sexuality out of the emotional, religious and guilt ridden context (which still persists) and opened way for objective research and discussion. Modern research workers such as Kinsey led investigations into normal sexual behaviour and Masters and Johnson developed techniques to overcome psychological bars to achieving satisfactory sexual responses leading to a more integrated personality.

Generally speaking, attitudes to sex learned from parents. Hence behaviour patterns tend to persist from one generation to another and change only slowly. Where facilities poor for education, communication, transport, traditional customs persist and are backed by authority. Where these facilities good, changes occur more quickly.

Sexual impulse

Evidence that libido affected by hormone levels especially

oestrogen in women and testosterone in men. However, major influence on libido is psychological and is a learned response. Great need in Western society for sex educators to teach people how best to react to their sexual drive without fear, disgust or guilt. Such educators need to be knowledgable, understanding, unbiased in any direction, highly ethical and unhampered by bigotry. Modern genèral practitioners of family medicine ideally placed to fulfil this role, though many unwilling because of their own ambivalent feeling about sex.

Many sexual hangups traced back to attitudes of shame, disgust, ignorance regarding body functions, especially those of opposite sex. When idea that human bodies are not dirty, indeed, the opposite, becomes accepted progress can be rapid.

Ideally, sexual interactions occur between two people and develop over a period of time in an environment free from hurry, worry and interference. Sexual act itself is only one part of mutual respect which should develop. Ultimately, in very best of situations, sex becomes a delight pervading all the interactions of a family unit and reaching peaks of physical union from time to time. Only in wider context of home and family can the heights of sexuality be reached. Where ideal situations cannot be achieved sexual satisfaction is less than perfect but still may be satisfactory.

Most common causes of female sexual dissatisfaction are premature ejaculation of male and failure to orgasm of female. These two often interwoven and interdependent. More likely to occur when partners fail to communicate with each other. Imperative that each partner knows what the other likes and does not like so that foreplay, i.e. stroking, fondling, caressing, kissing, can be effective in bringing both to brink of climax.

Easiest way to achieve satisfaction is to strive to give satisfaction to partner. To do so one must find out what partner wants which is an ongoing process. Premature ejaculation controlled by squeeze technique perfected by Masters and Johnson in which male indicates he is getting close to ejaculation and female then applies firm gentle pressure to glans. This causes disexcitation and some loss of erection and foreplay begins again, then penetration, back to almost ejaculation, withdrawal, squeeze and so on. Usually length of time before squeeze required increases and female comes closer to orgasm. In perfectly matched technique ejaculation and orgasm occur simultaneously.

Failure to orgasm very common problem. May be necessary to achieve orgasm by masturbation in first instance. May be self administered or by partner. Clitoris rubbed gently with well lubricated finger or vibrator or tongue (cunnilingus). If penis inserted from behind, clitoral region left free for masturbation during intercourse, a method found to be highly rewarding.

Many women achieve repeated orgasms if partner learns to retard ejaculation. Males loses erection after ejaculation and cannot regain it immediately.

Coitus during menstruation

Medically, no reason why coitus cannot occur during menstruation. Many women have maximum drive then and achieve greater pleasure, able to orgasm more frequently and more quickly. For the fastidious a vaginal douche and wearing of condom or diaphragm helps.

Coitus during pregnancy and following birth

Not contraindicated unless abortion threatened or habitual. After 37 weeks head usually engaged and coitus should stop. Post-partum coitus may be resumed when vaginal healing complete about 6 weeks.

Dyspareunia (painful coitus)

Causes. Local. Thick hymen may prevent penetration. Attempts painful. Hymen needs surgical incision and removal.

Vaginismus. Spasm of vaginal muscles. Always psychosomatic. Fear, guilt or ignorance to be overcome by re-education, by gentle, understanding, sympathetic therapist. Relaxation techniques, positive reinforcement therapy, introduction of vaginal dilators first by woman herself, later by sex partner or therapist. Help essential from partner, who must also be taught his role. Encourage lengthy foreplay, use lubricant, be unhurried and gentle.

Post-partum or post-surgical stenosis. May need dilation under general anaesthetic or vaginoplasty.

Vulvitis, Bartholinitis, vaginitis. Treat cause. Stop coitus until cured.

Post-menopausal atrophy. Apply oestrogen cream. Use lubricant jelly.

Deep dyspareunia

Experienced only on deep penetration or, rarely, after coitus is over.

Causes. Retroverted uterus, fibroids, oophoritis, salpingitis, pelvic inflammation, neoplasms of uterus, rectum, sigmoid colon.

Treatment. Careful pelvic examination to determine cause which is then treated.

Other sexual outlets

Where more usual forms of sexual expression denied to a woman she may achieve release from sexual tension by alternative methods.

No longer regarded as sexual deviations and their practitioners not regarded as abnormal but merely as people with needs that they fulfill as best they can under their circumstances.

To deny sexual pressure exists or to forbid any form of sexual outlet other than female/male intercourse is evidence of confused thinking. Many women have no opportunity to develop a sexual relationship with a suitable male partner but can nevertheless find satisfying sexual expression by fantasy building, masturbation or with another woman. Sensible attitude, understanding, and acceptance of their self-assessment needed. No place for condemnation and rejection.

Plight of disabled persons regarding sexuality recently receiving sympathetic attention. Again, understanding, advice and help necessary. Physical, skin to skin contact with another human being seems essential to mental and physical well being. How this can be arranged may be largely a matter for themselves but their need must be recognised and opportunities to meet others encouraged. Even when orgasm or erection or ejaculation impossible, a person may derive intense sexual satisfaction from bringing a partner to a climax.

Sex education

Best performed by parents by answering questions truthfully when asked and by setting example of personal affection towards partner. Many parents unwilling or unable to talk to their children because their own concepts are clouded with taboos, inhibitions, prejudices.

Sex education programmes in schools do not always meet needs of groups receiving them. Educator needs to be knowledgable, able to impart information without embarrassment, to be respected by the students and accepted by them. Often family physicians most suitable provided they view problems from point of view of the students and not from that which they held when they were students themselves.

7. Contraception

Definition
Prevention of pregnancy by preventing conception or preventing implantation.

Methods to keep sperm from ova
1. Coitus interuptus
2. Condom or sheath
3. Vaginal diaphragm or Dutch cap
4. Mini pill (progestogen only)
5. Rhythm or ovulation method
6. Tubal ligation

Methods to destroy sperm
1. Vaginal douche
2. Spermicidal creams or foams
3. Male pill
4. Vasectomy

Methods to suppress ovulation
1. Contraceptive pill

Methods to prevent implantation
1. Progestogens
2. Intra-uterine device

Coitus interuptus. Penis withdrawn just before male climax. High failure rate.

Unaesthetic. Great dissatisfaction psychologically and physiologically.

Condom or sheath. Thin rubber sheath placed over penis. Suitable lubricant, often spermicidal, renders it almost undetectable during coitus. Satisfactory if used properly. Interrupts spontaneity but putting it on can be made part of foreplay. Can become dislodged. May have holes in it if stored too long.

Vaginal diaphragm. Shallow rubber cup with spring loaded

circumferential rim. Extends from posterior fornix to behind symphysis pubis. Spermacidal jelly placed in cup before insertion so that cervix immersed. Can become dislodged. May have holes in it.

Mini-pill. Progestogen only. Norethisterone 0·35 mg taken daily. No breaks. Alters consistency of cervical mucus making it difficult for sperms to penetrate. No effect on ovulation. Slightly less reliable than other contraceptive pills.

Useful method for females in danger of thrombosis, who are lactating, or who are at climacteric age but still need contraception.

Rhythm method. Abstinence of coitus around time of ovulation. Very successful method if used by intelligent women. Time of ovulation established by carefully kept temperature charts extending over several cycles. Temperature taken at same time every day using same thermometer and same route, preferably rectal or vaginal. Rise in basal temperature is small 0·5 to 0·75° C. only. Careless recording can easily miss it. Once regular pattern established coitus stops from 3 days before expected day of ovulation to 4 days after actual day as determined by temperature. Method accepted by Roman Catholic prelate.

Disadvantages — ovulation may occur early, sperm may remain active for 48 hours.

Tubal ligation. Fallopian tubes ligated and usually sectioned. Prevents passage of sperm towards ovum and passage of ova to uterus. Disadvantages — introduces dangers of general anaesthetic and opening abdomen. May be done via laparoscope under local anaesthetic. Tubes cauterised but not tied. Damage to other organs possible by this method.

Tubal ligation usually regarded as irreversible but some success recently with excision of obliterated ends and anastomosis under operating microscope vision.

Vaginal douche. Effective in cleaning out vagina if carried out within seconds of coitus. Spermicidal douches used — vinegar, quinine, lead acetate. Method totally ineffective in removing sperm already through cervix. If satisfactory orgasm occurs uterus exerts powerful suction effect which draws semen through cervix.

Spermicidal creams. Many substances very effective in

rendering sperm immobile in laboratory, but mixing semen with cream inside vagina far from effective especially if male climax and female orgasm occur simultaneously and semen immediately aspirated. Best used inside condom or diaphragm.

Male 'pill'. Experiments proceeding to suppress spermatogenesis without interfering with production of testosterone. Not yet ready for use on humans.

Vasectomy. Removal of sections of vasa deferentia and ligation. (Male tubal ligation.) Performed through small incisions in scrotum. Highly successful form of contraception. Spermatogenis stops but testosterone production continues. Irreversible, hence recipient must be quite sure he does not want more children. Does not reduce libido or male performance. Quantity of semen reduced slightly.

Contraceptive pill (O.C.'s)

Most commonly used. Estimated between 50 and 100 million users throughout world. Combination of ethinyl oestradiol or mestranol with one of six or seven progestogens. Pill taken for 21 days and then stopped for 7 days (or non-pill taken for 7 days).

Sequential pill supplies oestrogen only for 15 days then oestrogen plus progestogen for 5 days.

Resembles normal physiological pattern of hormone production. No sequential pills available as such in Australia but regime can be prescribed using ethinyl oestradiol and norethisterone tablets if sequential regime required for some reason, e.g. irregular menstruation.

All common combination O.C.'s contain either 30 μg or 50 μg or 100μg oestrogen. Dosage of progestogen depends on potency of particular one.

Giving medroxyprogesterone acetate arbitrary potency of 1 unit remaining common ones can be arranged in comparable scale:

Norethisterone 1.3
Megestrol acetate 2
Norethisterone acetate 2.7
Lynestrenol 2.7

Chlormadinone 20
Etynodiol diacetate 20
D, 1 – Norgestrel 40
D, – Norgestrel 80

Hence, the combination most suited to particular women can be chosen from about 20 various groupings.

Actions. All combination O.C.'s suppress pituitary output of releasing hormone and FSH and LH production. Hence ovulation fails.

Other actions. Progestogen alters cervical mucus making it thick and impenetrable to sperm. Endometrium altered making it less suitable for implantation. Tubal transport interfered with.

Complications. Combination pill has widespread effects on all tissues, some apparently harmless, others potentially lethal. As far as possible doctor prescribing pill originally should exclude conditions known to be associated with complications and should check users at least annually to ensure continued health.

'Harmless' side effects. Nausea, vomiting, headache, leucorrhoea, chloasma, breast enlargement and tenderness, intermenstrual spotting.

'Beneficial' side effects. Pain-free periods, diminished menstrual loss, predictable timing of periods, breast enlargement (in some cases), reduced severity of acne, increased libido, relief from pre-menstrual tension.

Serious complications

Thrombo-embolic disorders — deep vein thrombosis (DVT), cerebral embolism. Risk of DVT increased five times from 0·02 to 0·1 per cent of women at risk. Risk of cerebral embolism increased four times from 0·01 to 0·04 per cent of women at risk.

Risk is related to dose of oestrogen and hence low dose pill preferred. Other factors may increase thrombo-embolic risk, e.g. smoking, increasing age (three times greater over 35 years) surgical operations, raised blood pressure, diabetes mellitus, presence of varicose veins. Great care needed before initiating oral contraceptives in women with these risk factors.

Hypertension. Some women show marked rise in both systolic and diastolic pressures. Ninety-five per cent of users show no increase after 5 years of use. Probably sensible to restrict use among those already suffering from hypertension and among older women with family history of hypertension.

Liver disorders. Steroids known to hinder enzymes concerned with excretion of bile. In normal women low dose contraceptive pill unlikely to cause noticeable change but in those with history of liver disease or jaundice during pregnancy should not be prescribed oestrogens.

Diseases linked to O.C.'s include cholestatic jaundice, benign hepatoma (31 cases recorded), increased gall stone formation.

Diabetes mellitus. Alteration of glucose tolerance noted in 15 to 40 per cent of women on O.C.'s. Contraindicated in those with frank diabetes and great care needed in obese, over 35's or those with family history of diabetes.

Depression. Depressive illness may arise soon after starting O.C.'s and disappear when stopped. Difficult to obtain 'pure' evidence to state unequivocally that cause is simply O.C.'s. However, incidence less on low dose oestrogens though psychological effect of the reassuring doctor may have as much to do with reduced incidence.

Fetal abnormalities. No firm evidence that O.C.'s linked to congenital abnormalities, but some evidence incriminating progestogens when used as pregnancy tests, and when progesterone was used to prevent abortion. Reported to be higher incidence of early spontaneous abortion when taking O.C.'s but refuted by other researchers. However, use of O.C.'s and especially mini-pill (progestogen only), ceased if pregnancy does occur and termination not contemplated.

Cancer. No evidence for increased risk of breast, uterine or cervical cancer with O.C.'s. Indeed, recent research suggests O.C.'s give some protection against occurence of gynaecological cancer and of non-malignant breast tumours.

Female offspring of mothers who had stilboestrol therapy during early pregnancy to prevent abortion sometimes develop vaginal cancer at puberty. Rare, unusual, and stilboestrol never used for such purpose now.

Post-pill amenorrhoea. A few women fail to menstruate when O.C. stopped. More likely to occur if: (1) started menstruating late 16 to 18 years of age; (2) periods always scanty prior to starting O.C.; (3) cycle always irregular; (4) thin, boyish, small breasted figure with problem of acne. Patient should be reassured that menstruation will start again. If none after 6 months ovulation stimulated with chlomiphene citrate.

Prevention of side effects and complications

Risks with all drugs. These must always be weighed against beneficial effects if doctor prescribing O.C.'s takes care to weed out as far as possible, those running high risk of complications, and keep on assessing users as years go by, risks reduced to minimum. In Australia prescription limited to 6 month's supply. Women should always be assessed before renewal of script and not given new script as a routine.

Initial assessment should include menstrual history, past history of hypertension, diabetes, jaundice, thrombosis, breast lumps, varicose veins, migraine headaches, epilepsy, examination of blood pressure, breasts, cervix, cervical smear for cervical cancer, urine test for albumen and sugar.

Six monthly check should include blood pressure, breast examination, questioning for side effects, and follow up for these.

Two yearly cervical smears reducing to 6 monthly if dysplasia occurs followed by cone biopsy if necessary.

Women advised to reduce risk factors to minimum — stop smoking, keep weight to normal level, stop O.C.'s when family size satisfactory and choose tubal ligation or vasectomy.

Other forms of oral contraception

'Morning after' contraception. Midcycle coitus particularly likely to cause pregnancy when no precautions taken. To avoid this a 5 day course of ethinyl oestradiol should be started within 72 hours but preferably within 24 hours.

Dose and regime:

Stemetil 5 mg 8 a.m. and 8 p.m.

Ethinyl oestradiol tabs 0·5 mg × 2 at 9 a.m.

Ethinyl oestradiol tabs 0·5 mg × 3 at 9 p.m.

Continue for 5 days.

High dose of ethinyl oestradiol causes nausea and may cause vomiting hence need for stemetil.

Very successful but very nauseating. Best reserved for cases of rape or incest.

Once-a-month pill. Not yet perfected but promising results from (a) quinestrol, a new long acting oestrogen absorbed from intestine, stored in body fat depots and slowly released over a month, and (b) combination quinestrol and quingestonon pill, a new progestogen.

Disadvantages — unreliable absorption from intestine, uneven release from fat depots, hence insufficient control over action.

Annual subcutaneous implant. In use in South America, India and Scandinavia. Small incision in forearm allows implant of either silastic rod or silastic capsule.

Rod 3 cm long 2·4 mm wide (inch by $\frac{1}{10}$ inch approx.) impregnated with 40 mg D-norgestrol, silastic capsule filled with D-norgestrel. The progestogen slowly releases from rod or leaks out of capsule in sufficient amount to antagonise oestrogen feedback on pituitary, hence gonadotrophin secretion reduced and ovulation fails.

Disadvantages — breakthrough bleeding unpredictable. Usually minor spotting but may be prolonged. No regular menstrual pattern. Present aim— to improve absorption and achieve amenorrhoea. Special implement needed for insertion. Norgestrel may cause increased growth of facial hair and acne.

Advantages— once a year attention. Action reversed when implant removed or wears out.

8. Climacteric

Climacteric refers to changes occuring in anatomy, physiology and psyche when reproductive life ends.

Menopause refers to cessation of menstruation. Both terms generally used interchangeably. Often term 'change of life' used.

Age of onset

Round about 46 years of age. As early as 40. Rarely later than 52. Depends on ovarian output. Occurs at any age if ovaries removed or destroyed, e.g. by radiation or by interference with blood supply during hysterectomy.

Adverse symptoms

Vasomotor disturbance causes hot flushes, excessive sweating, headaches, fainting spells and palpitations.

Menstruation may cease abruptly. More commonly periods become irregular. May be scanty or increased and then stop.

Skin becomes coarser, dryer, loses elasticity and may start wrinkling.

Vulval atrophy commences. Dryness may cause dyspareunia.

Bodily changes. Breasts — may be some increase in fat initially. Later reabsorption of fat leaving breasts flat. Nipples diminish and flatten.

Vulva and vagina. Absorption of fat within labia majora, loss of rugae from vaginal mucosa, diminished vagina secretion. Loss of normal acidity. Changes encourage trauma and infection.

Uterus. Gradually atrophy of muscle, cervix, endometrium.

Bones. Some demineralisation common. In some cases osteoporosis very marked causing severe backache, spontaneous collapse fractures of vertebral bodies, fragility of all bones making fractures common from minor trauma. Cause not known but administration of oestrogen diminishes tendency to fracture. Other treatment — calcium 1 g daily, vitamin D 1000 units daily, sodium fluoride 20 mg daily. Maintain mobility and activity supervised by physiotherapist.

Heart and vessels. Some evidence that vascular system protected by oestrogen. Incidence of atherosclerosis, coronary antery disease, hypertension, lower in women than men up to age 50 then closing of gap as age advances.

Psychological. Depression, insomnia, lassitude, commonly occur. Whether due to alterations in hormone balance or to other changes occuring at this time of life is not clear, e.g. reduction in family demands, sporting participation, fading of ambitions, changing social role, slower pace of life. Libido usually unaltered but may increase (20 per cent) or decrease (20 per cent).

Adjustment of climacteric goes through three phases:
1. Impact. Realisation that fertility has ceased may cause anxiety about sexuality and desirability
2. Recoil, or denial. Mood changes, depression, irritability common. Occasionally women become hyperactive taking part in sports, games, social activities. Alcoholism may become problem
3. Readjustment. Amost all women finally accept new image.

Hormonal changes. Diminishing output of oestrogen which may fluctuate as long as responsive tissue remains in ovary. No progesterone once ovulation stops. Adrenal continues very low oestrogen output until old age.

Gonadotrophins increase to tenfold pre-menopausal level and remain high until old age.

Adrenal output of all steroids decline very slowly.

Treatment. Most women require no active treatment. Explanation, support and reassurance that they are not becoming ugly, useless and unwanted and sympathetic easing through a difficult time is needed.

Occasionally a mild anxiolytic helpful but some danger of psychological dependence developing. Diazepam 2 mg or oxazepam 15 mg nightly to be reviewed monthly. Occasionally depressive illness is severe and needs full antidepressive measures — tricyclic anti-depressants, e.g. amitriptylline, up to 150 mg daily.

Symptomatic relief of frequent hot flushes by oestrogen

therapy. Low daily dose at first. Ethinyl oestradiol 0·01–0·05 mg for 3 weeks each month. May need to increase up to 0·1–0·2 mg until flushes reduced to bearable minimum. Alternately equine conjugated oestrogen used (Premarin), 0·625 mg daily for 3 weeks each month.

Older forms of hormone therapy no longer advised — oestrogen/progesterone combination, stilboestrol, androgens.

9. Venereal Diseases

Definition
Diseases which are transmitted by sexual contact.
Gonorrhoea
Syphilis
Lymphogranuloma inguinale
Granuloma venereum
Some authorities include haemophilis vaginalis, monilia, trichomonas infection, pubic lice and scabies among venereal diseases.

Gonorrhoea

Cause. Gram-negative diplococcus. Neisseria gonorrhoeae. Delicate organism dying easily outside body. Penetrates into moist surface of vulva, vagina, cervix, urethra, ducts of Bartholin's and Skene's glands.
Incubation period. 2 to 10 days.
Acute signs and symptoms. Pain on micturition. Purulent discharge from urethra and vagina. Sore, tender swollen vulva and vagina. May be severe general symptoms of toxaemia — temperature, malaise, joint and muscle aches.
On examination, vulvitis, vaginitis, cervicitis, copious pus.
Diagnosis. Gram stain of freshly made smear shows diplococci within pus cells. Culture on special medium grows typical colonies.
Smears should be taken from cervical canal, vaginal wall and urethral orifice, fixed immediately and examined as soon as possible. If delayed before reaching laboratory swabs immersed in Stuart's transport medium.

Chronic disease
If untreated, local acute symptoms generally subside but organisms migrate to fallopian tubes, peritoneum, anal

mucosa or may be blood borne to joints.. Those in Bartholin's and Skene's glands and ducts remain as continuous source of infection.

Treatment. Acute gonorrhoea usually responds to single injection procaine penicillin 1 g i.m. In some regions penicillin resistant strains emerging needing treatment with cotrimoxazole (Septrin, Bactrim, Trib) two tablets b.i.d. for 10 days or tetracycline 500 mg q.i.d. for 10 days.

Chronic gonorrhoea often intractable needing treatment with other antibiotics, e.g. cephalosporin, gentamycin, Kanamycin or streptomycin. Main complication of gonorrhoea is chronicity in female causing salpingitis, peritonitis and sterility.

Syphilis

Cause. Spirochaete, Treponema pallidum. Corkscrew-like organism able to bore through intact skin and mucosa. Living organism may be seen with dark ground illumination in fresh specimen.

Incubation period. Ten to 90 days, most commonly 14 to 28.

Pathology. If untreated, disease passes through three stages. Primary: secondary: tertiary.

Primary manifestations. Small papule grows at site of penetration of organism, usually on vulva but may be vagina, cervix, anus, lip. Papule breaks down to shallow painless ulcer with sharply defined edge and surrounded by area of hard induration. Hence usual name — hard chancre.

Regional lymph nodes, usually inguinal, become hard but do not break down. This stage easily missed and healing takes place within 2 to 3 weeks.

Secondary manifestations. General — temperature, malaise; skin rash — coppery spots over chest, abdomen and anterior aspect of forearms; May mimic any type of rash. Non irritant. Fades without trace. Other more rare symptoms are alopecia, mouth ulcers, iritis, generalised adenitis.

Tertiary stage. Organisms cause thickening and obliteration of arterioles anywhere in body. Infarction at various sites — skin causing painless ulcers — gumma; bone — erosions; brain — general paralysis of the insane; spinal cord — tabes dorsalis; aorta — aneurysm.

Diagnosis. Organism recovered from pus at base of primary chancre.

Serological tests numerous. Commonly used — VDRL (Venereal Diseases Research Laboratory) test because it becomes positive early in disease, Wasserman, Kline, Kahn tests are complement fixation tests positive about 6 weeks after infection. Fluorescent Treponema antibody test and Treponema immobilisation test, are highly specific for syphilis.

Treatment. Procaine penicillin 1 g daily for 10 days.

Dangers. Danger of non-treatment is progression to insanity or crippling deformity. Organism can be passed via placenta to fetus.

Lymphogranuloma inguinale

Cause. Chlamydia. Similar organism to that causing psittacosis and trachoma. Causes meningitis in mice and monkeys.

Distribution. World wide but especially prevalent in tropical areas.

Incubation period. Two to 30 days.

Signs and symptoms. Small shallow painless ulcer on external genitalia. May be missed easily and patient first complains of hard lumps in inguinal and femoral regions. Regional lymph nodes become hard, swollen, matted together. Abscess breaks down forming multiple sinuses. In female upper vaginal lymphatics drain to rectal lymph nodes which enlarge similarly.

Blood borne organisms may cause, meningitis, pericarditis, conjunctivitis, arthritis, skin lesions.

Untreated, lymphadenitis causes obstruction and elephantiasis of genitalia, chronic abscesses, stricture of rectum.

Diagnosis. Complement fixation test on serum. Skin reaction test (Frei's test) indicates infection at some time but does not necessarily indicate present disease.

Treatment. Tetracycline 500 mg q.i.d. for 30 days.

Granuloma venereum

Cause. Bacillus, Donovania granulomatis.

Distribution. World wide but more common in tropics.

Incubation periods. Three to 40 days.

Signs and symptoms. Well defined painless ulcer which spreads slowly to form large sore with granulating red base. Easily mistaken for cancer when occuring on cervix. Organism may spread to bones, joints, viscera.

Diagnosis. Identification of organisms lying in large mononuclear cells in scrapings from base of ulcer or biopsy of edge.

Difficult to establish diagnosis in chronic cases.

Treatment. Tetracycline 500 mg q.i.d. for 15 days.

10. The Vulva

Anatomy

External genitalia— mons veneris, labia majora, labia minora, clitoris, urethral meatus, hymen, vestibule, Bartholin's glands, Skene's glands.

Mons veneris. Skin overlying fat pad covering pubic bones.

Labia majora. Two skin folds bearing hair covering fat pads, between mons superiorly and perineum inferiorly.

Labia minora. Two modified skin folds between labia majora. Fat free, hair free. Abundant sebaceous glands. Unite superiorly to form hood or prepuce surrounding clitoris. Unite inferiorly to form posterior commissure or fourchette. Large in children and protrude between labia majora. Atrophic in menopause.

Clitoris. Female counterpart of penis. Small, highly sensitive organ. Has all the parts of penis in miniature, glans covered by hood or prepuce, erectile tissue — corpora cavernosa attached to pubic rami, vestibular bulbs one on each side surrounding introitus. Corpora cavernosa and vestibular bulbs of erectile tissue. Clitoral stimulation either directly, or secondarily from tension through vestibular bulbs during intercourse leads to reflex orgasm.

Urethral meatus. External opening of urethra.

Hymen. Membranous layer partly closing vagina. Occasionally imperforate (see page 26). Ruptures at first coitus. Remnants form line of tags called carunculae myrtiformes.

Vestibule. That part of the opening lying between the labia minora with the clitoris above and the vagina below.

Bartholin's glands. One on each side buried in tissue between labia majora and minora. Secrete mucus to lubricate introitus before coitus.

Skene's glands. One on each side of urethral meatus. Several small ducts, Skene's tubules, conduct secretion to meatus.

Blood supply. Internal pudendal arteries from internal iliac arteries supply almost all structures. External pudendal arteries from femoral arteries supply parts of labia and mons veneris.

Veins accompany arteries. Few drain to long saphenous.

Lymphatics. Important when considering spread of carcinoma. Superficial network unites with that of anterior abdominal wall. Pass through superficial inguinal glands to deep inguinal and deep femoral then to external iliac to join net from deeper structures at internal iliac glands.

Nerves. Sensory derived from lumbar plexus via ilio-inguinal nerves to mons and anterior vulval structures, genital branch of genito-femoral to labia, posterior cutaneous nerve of thigh to perineum and labia. Also from sacral plexus via pudendal nerves to clitoris and deeper vulval structures. Also supplies motor nerves to urethra, levator ani and anal sphincter.

Conditions affecting the vulva

Pruritis vulvae

Very common symptom. Sometimes persistent and severe.

Causes

1. Local. 75 per cent monilia or trichomonas infection. Allergies and sensitivities to soaps, sprays, plastics in clothing, parasites — crab lice, scabies. Aspect of skin condition: eczema, lichen planus, psoriasis. Vulval dystrophy, dysplasia and cancer
2. General diseases. Diabetes. Deficiencies: vitamin B, folic acid, iron. Menopausal atrophy. Psychosomatic.

Investigations. Careful history. (In children vulvo-vaginitis most common gynaecological problem. Frequently in association with nose, throat, ear, infections.)

General examination where indicated.

Local examination for extent of irritation, discharge, excoriation, parasites. Laboratory tests. Urine for infection, sugar.

Vaginal swabs for fresh wet smears to detect trichomonas and/or monilia (candida). Swabs for gonorrhoea if this is suspected.

Blood for syphilis.

Biopsy of skin if precancerous or cancerous lesion suspected.

Treatment. Depends on cause. Diabetic control. Antibiotics
for VD's. Metronidazole for trichomonas. Nystatin cream or
pessaries for monilia. Povidine iodine for non specific infections. Oestrogen creams for post-menopausal atrophy. Generally — improvement of hygiene. Pre-cancerous and cancerous lesions — vulvectomy, irradiation (see page 116).

Vulval infections

Usually associated with vaginal infections. In childhood and
post-menopause, lack of oestrogen allows many common
organisms to flourish. In children labia minora more exposed.
Often infection localised, transient and not associated with
vaginitis. Many organisms responsible. Trichomonas, monilia,
streptococcus, staphylococcus, diphtheria, gonoccocus,
spirochaeta pallidum.

Signs and symptoms. Pain worse while sitting or walking.
Burning on micturition. Itch. Labia inflamed, tender, swollen.
Pus or discharge. Pressure below urethral meatus may reveal
pus. Pressure over Bartholin's glands similarly. May be
general symptoms pyrexia, weakness, toxaemia.

Investigations. Swabs taken for culture and sensitivity. Wet
smears examined for trichomonas and monilia.

Treatment. Immediate palliative: rest in bed, sitz bath,
bathe vulva with mild antiseptic, apply soothing antiseptic
cream, e.g. Savlon.

Specific: Nystatin cream for monilia, metronidazole for
trichomonas, penicillin for streptococcal, gonococcal or
syphilitic infection. Antibiotic according to sensitivity for
others.

Non-specific: povidine iodine.

Condylomata acuminata

Warts from viral infection. Often accompany VD's but not
necessarily. Spread by sexual intercourse.

Diagnosis. By inspection. Warty growths of varying size
from 0·5 to 10 mm diameter. May be very extensive covering
entire vulva. Rarely invade far into vagina. May involve anus.

Treatment. If few and small, diathermy under local
anaesthetic or application of 20 per cent podophyllin in oil.
Care needed to avoid normal skin. Allowed to dry. Washed

off after 8 hours. Warts shrivel and separate within 10 days. May need second or more applications.

Urethral caruncle

Small, very painful polyp arising from mucous membrane of urethra. Almost always associated with senile atrophy.

Cause. Probably chronic infection of meatus.

Signs and symptoms. Pain on passing urine. Tender area in vestibule. Bright red mass at urethral meatus usually posteriorly. Usually granulomatous, occasionally glandular or vascular.

Treatment. Excision, cautery of base, treat urinary infection. Recurrent caruncles should be biopsied for malignancy.

Urethral prolapse

May be confused with caruncle but close examination shows prolapse to be a concentric protrusion of mucous membrane round meatus and not a discrete lump.

Signs and symptoms. Acute: pain, frequency, dysuria. Dark red swelling round meatus. Chronic: gaping meatus. Usually painless but liable to ulceration.

Treatment. Acute: replace mucous membrane. Insert indwelling catheter until oedema and swelling subside. Excise prolapsing mucous membrane.

Chronic: apply antiseptic creams or paints, e.g. povidine iodine. When oedema subsides encourage epithelialisation with oestrogen cream. Excise if necessary.

Bartholinitis

Definition. Infection of Bartholin's ducts and/or glands.

Causative organisms. Streptococci, staphylococci, gonococci.

Signs and symptoms. Painful, red, swollen, hot lump, starting just inside labium minus posteriorly. Surrounding cellulitis and oedema may make examination painful and difficult.

Treatment. Rest in bed, antibiotics, analgesics. Incise and drain if resolution fails to occur. If cyst or chronic abscess develops, de-roof and marsupialise.

Cysts

Three types occur. Bartholin's. Sebaceous. Gartner's.

1. Bartholin's. Single, rounded swelling posteriorly. Rarely more than 3 cm diameter. Painless unless infected. May cause dyspareunia.

Treatment. Marsupialisation.

2. Sebaceous. May occur anywhere on hair bearing areas or on labia minora. Any size from 1 mm to 3 cm. Usually painless unless infected.

Treatment. Excision.

3. Gartner's cyst. Forms along line of remnant of embryological structure — mesonephric duct. Cyst may appear near clitoris, hymen, labia minora. Usually small — up to 1 cm — painless. May disappear on pressure. No treatment unless causing dyspareunia.

Ulceration

Occur anywhere on vulva.

Causes. Trauma, Infection. Malignancy. More likely to occur in post-menopause.

Organisms. Tubercle bacillus, spirochaeta pallidum, herpes virus, organisms of specific infectious diseases. Non-specific secondary invaders. Organisms of lymphogranuloma inguinale and granuloma venereum.

Treatment. Biopsy to exclude malignancy (see page 56). Specific antibiotics when organisms identified. Bathing and application of antiseptics if traumatic.

New growths

May be benign or malignant.

Benign:

Hidradenoma, tumour arising from sweat gland

Lipoma — fatty tumour

Fibroma and fibromyoma of labia

Papilloma. Suspicious post-menopausal.

Malignant:

Carcinoma

Squamous cell carcinoma. Most common. 95 per cent

Basal cell carcinoma

Adenocarcinoma. Associated with Bartholin's gland

Melanoma.

Presentation. Benign tumours usually present with painless lump in young woman.

Malignant tumours present with either lump or ulcer or

change of skin texture, almost always over 55 years of age. Occasionally frank cauliflower-like mass.

Pre-malignant conditions

Carcinoma almost always preceded by intractable, long standing pruritis.

Skin may be atrophic, pale, shiny, ulcerates readily. Or may be red, thickened, with white patches in moist areas — leukoplakia.

Chronic vulval epithelial dystrophies require biopsy. Atrophic pattern shows thinning of epidermis and loss of rete pegs. In hypertrophic pattern show thickening and exaggeration of rete pegs.

Dysplasia shown by thickened, dense epithelial cells with crowding and irregularity of basal cells, long irregular rete pegs, hyalinisation in sub-epithelial zone and loss of elastic fibres.

Investigations. Biopsy from several points around vulva, labia majora and minora.

If ulcer or lump present biopsy taken to include edge of ulcer and part of lump adjoining normal skin.

Treatment. Atrophic and hypetrophic vulvae — conservative with strict attention to hygiene, sitz baths, antiseptics, oestrogen cream, regular inspection to note any change.

Dysplasia with no invasion of dermis, vulvectomy without lymphadenectomy.

Carcinoma — radical vulvectomy.

All vulval skin removed with extensive margin extending to anterior superior iliac spines and femoral triangles laterally, from anal margin to symphysis pubis, and include labia minora internally, Superficial inguinal nodes taken. Follow up at 6 monthly intervals for rest of life.

Staging. Treatment rests on degree to which cancer has progressed.

Stage 0. Microscopic evidence of malignancy confined to epidermis. Simple vulvectomy

Stage I. Area involved limited to 5 sq. cm with no spread. Radical vulvectomy

Stage II. Area greater than 5 sq. cm or spread locally to anus, urethra or vagina but not to glands

Stage III. Nodes involved

Stage IV. Extensive spread to rectum, bone, bladder or evidence of metastases

Stages III and IV have very poor prognosis. May be treated by simple vulvectomy for symptomatic improvement or by irradiation or both.

11. The Vagina

Anatomy

Fibromuscular tube extending from vulva to cervix between urethra and bladder in front and rectum and pouch of Douglas behind. Similar pocket of peritoneum separates bladder and vagina but is very variable in extent. Laterally, ureters cross upper vaginal walls on way to bladder.

Superiorly, cervix projects in anterior wall of vagina. Areas surrounding cervix called fornices (sing. fornix) anterior, two lateral and deep posterior fornix. Access to pouch of Douglas and peritoneal cavity readily achieved via posterior fornix — colpotomy, culdoscopy.

Vaginal walls consist of three layers — outer, muscular subdivided into two, external continuous with myometrium, internal of voluntary fibres from levator ani which encircle introitus to form a sphincter; middle layer of connective tissue; lining of stratified squamous epitheluim.

Lining epitheluim undergoes changes in thickness and secretion depending on levels of circulating oestrogen. Deepest layer — rounded basal cells forming conical projections deep into fibrous layer called rete pegs. Next, several layers of rounded parabasal cells, then several layers of flattened intermediate cells. Lastly surface layers of flattened large area cells with small central nucleus. With plentiful oestrogen intermediate and superficial cells numerous, fast growing, contain much glycogen. Stain dark brown with iodine — an important test for malignant change (see page 74).

Physiology

Vaginal walls kept moist mainly by cervical secretions but partly by transudation through epithelium. Transudation increases in sexual excitement during stage of hyperaemia of anticipation.

Glycogen content of epithelium encourages growth of lactobacillus (Doderlein's bacillus) which converts sugars to lactic acid causing reaction to be acid. Many other commensal organisms reside in vagina, staphylococci, streptococci, monilia, enterococci. Of no consequence during fertile years but may be cause of infection when acidity falls, e.g. when oestrogen absent before menarche or post-menopause. When oral contraceptives used, epithelium rich in glycogen and monilia may flourish then.

Development

Vagina develops from two sources, down-growing Mullerian ducts fuse to form uterus and upper 4/5 of vagina, upgrowing urogenital sinus forms vulva and lower 1/5 of vagina. However, the lining epithelium is formed by ingrowth of cells from urogenital sinus — modified skin cells. These meet columnar cells growing down to line uterus at the external os of cervix— an important line of junction (see page 74).

Blood supply. Rich arterial supply from branches of uterine, internal pudendal, middle and inferior rectal arteries. Plexus of veins take blood back to internal iliac veins.

Lymphatics. Lower drain with vulval vessels to inguinal nodes, upper parts to rectal and pelvic nodes with cervical vessels.

Vaginal discharge

At birth newborn girl may have copious watery or bloodstained vaginal discharge due to oestrogen influence. Until menarche, vaginal discharge of any sort unusual. May indicate infection commonly from foreign body. At menarche cervical secretion moistens vaginal walls amount varying with oestrogen levels. Usually insufficient to escape from vulva but occasionally may do so when oestrogen level highest about time of ovulation.

If discharge is not due to infection termed leucorrhoea. May distress some women. May cause irritation. May be controlled with acidifying agent, e.g. Tampovagan lactic acid pessaries.

Discharge with foul odour or causing intense irritation or inflammation — sign of infection. Swabs needed to establish cause and sensitivity.

Blood-stained discharge other than menses should always be investigated. Usually coming from uterus. When derived from cervix or vagina, suggestive of cancer and must be investigated.

Infections

Vaginitis most common childhood gynaecological condition, usually but not necessarily involving vulva also — vulvo-vaginitis.

Causes in childhood:
1. Non specific
2. Monilia
3. Foreign body
4. Streptococcus
5. Staphylococcus
6. Trichomonas
7. Gonococcus

Causes in adults:
1. Monilia
2. Trichomonas
3. Non-specific
4. Gonorrhoea
5. Senile

Moniliasis (candidiasis, vaginal thrush)

Cause. Monilia albicans (Candida albicans). Yeast. Growth factors: warmth; moisture; acid medium; glycogen (or glucose in diabetes). Absence of competitors following recent anti-biotic course. Flares up if temperature raised as in systemic infections, and when oestrogen levels highest, e.g. in pregnancy or while taking combination oral contraceptives.

Signs and symptoms. Thick white granular discharge. Moderate to severe vulvo-vaginitis. Dyspareunia. Severe pruritis. Vaginal walls have numerous grey-white patches which bleed on removal.

Diagnosis. Fresh wet smear shows thread like hyphae. Stain readily Gram-positive. Cultures grow readily at room temperature on Nickerson's medium.

Treatment. Nystatin or natamycin pessaries or vaginal

cream inserted to vault of vagina twice daily for 10 days. Oral nystatin tablets may be used for repeated infections if bowel is suspected as source. Sexual partner may need local treatment to penis.

Urine test to exclude diabetes.

In children cream preferable. Inserted via small catheter attached to tube.

Trichomoniasis

Cause. Single cell protozoon, trichomonas vaginalis. Very large, 15 to 20 μm, highly motile, pear shaped with undulating membrane and four flagellae. Lives on cellular debris. Flourishes on red blood cells hence may flare up during menstruation. (Contrast monilia which flares up between periods.)

Incidence. Rare before puberty and post-menopausally. Very common during fertile years. Frequently lurks in male urethra, seminal vesicles, prepuce, without causing symptoms but reinfecting female during coitus.

Signs and symptoms. Copious greeny-white frothy discharge with offensive odour. Pruritis severe. Vulvo-vaginitis, dysuria, dyspareunia.

Diagnosis. Fresh, wet slide diluted with normal saline reveals organisms swimming about actively. Tiny amount of cotton wool under cover slip traps organism making it easier to see.

Treatment. Metronidazole (Flagyl) oral tablets 200 mg 1 t.i.d. for 7 days. Best given to both partners. Local applications: di-iodohydroxyquinoline (Floraquine) pessaries 1 night and morning, 10 days; Amphotericin (Fungilin); similarly Miconazole cream (gyno-Daktarin) nightly for 2 weeks.

Non-specific vaginitis

May be associated with trauma, lack of hygiene, foreign body, malignant tumour, allergy, diabetes.

Signs and symptoms. Pruritis, discharge which may be foul smelling ('lost' tampon), scalding on passing urine, dyspareunia. Inflammation.

Diagnosis. Look for foreign body. Exclude diabetes, malignant tumour or ulcer. Take swabs for culture and sensitivity to exclude specific organisms.

Treatment. Treat cause if found. Give antibiotic for

secondary invaders. Apply local antiseptics, e.g. povidine iodine 10 per cent. Improve general health and hygiene.

Gonorrhoea
See page 47.

Senile vaginitis
Cause. Lowered vitality and resistance due to atrophy, lack of oestrogens, reduced blood supply, alkaline reaction.

Signs and symptoms. As for non-specific vaginitis.

Diagnosis. Imperative to exclude carcinoma.

Treatment. Acid douches. Local application of antiseptics and oestrogen cream. Oral ethinyl oestradiol 0·01 mg, b.d.

Vaginal malformations
1. Absent vagina. Either in conjunction with absent uterus and tubes (developmental failure of Mullerian duct system) or with uterus and tubes present (developmental failure of urogenital sinus).

2. Septate vagina. Mullerian ducts fail to fuse wholly leaving membrane. Rarely two complete vaginae associated with two uteri.

3. Transverse septa. Incomplete canalisation of solid mass following fusion of Mullerian ducts.

4. Imperforate hymen. Failure of fusion between urogenital sinus and Mullerian ducts.

Diagnosis. Usually delayed until menarche when amenorrhoea or cryptomenorrhoea occurs (see page 26) or difficulty with sexual intercourse.

Treatment. Septa divided. Hymen excised. New vagina fashioned when absent, using strip of skin from thigh fashioned into tube and inserted into space made by separating layers between bladder and rectum. (Maclude-Read operation) or epithelium from labia minora utilised (William's operation.)

Fistulae of vagina
Vagina may communicate with urethra, bladder or ureter anteriorly or with anus, rectum or colon posteriorly.

Causes. Almost always traumatic, from birth injury, surgery or irradiation. Occasionally from infection, e.g. tuberculosis, lymphogranuloma inguinale, or complicating carcinoma of any organ in vicinity.

Diagnosis. Incontinent passage of urine or faeces from vagina. Insertion methylene blue into rectum or bladder stains tampon in vagina. Ureterovaginal fistula needs retrograde pyelography to locate side and site.

Treatment. Urethrovaginal. Simple closure round catheter left in situ until healed. Suprapubic cystotomy may be necessary.

Vesicovaginal. Suprapubic cystotomy and/or catheter drainage with antiseptic washouts and antibiotics until healthy tissues present then closure surgically.

Ureterovaginal. If low down, ureter divided and replanted into bladder. If high up may be necessary to perform nephrectomy. Occasionally excision of fistula and anastomosis of ureter possible.

Anovaginal. Bowel prepared with antibiotic cover. Fistula closed from both sides, anal and vaginal.

Rectovaginal. Similar but may need temporary colostomy to allow healing.

Vaginocolic. Rare. Usually complicating carcinoma. Colostomy usually controls.

Urethral diverticulum
Congenital or secondary to urethritis.

Signs and symptoms. Midline swelling of anterior vaginal wall, frequent urinary tract infections.

Diagnosis. Micturating cysto-urethrogram.

Treatment. Surgical excision. Allow healing round catheter.

Genital prolapse
Causes. Weakness of vaginal walls, stretching of muscles of pelvic floor, late sequel of childbirth, ageing of tissues.

Types. Urethrocele. Urethra bulges into anterior vagina.

Cystocele. Bladder bulges into anterior vagina.

Rectocele. Rectum bulges into posterior vagina.

Enterocele. Loops of sigmoid colon or small intestine bulge into posterior vagina via pouch of Douglas.

Uterine prolapse (see page 69).

Commonly, various combinations occur.

Signs and symptoms. Vaginal lump noticed. Urinary tract

infection more likely, because of incomplete emptying, causing frequency, dysuria, urgency. Stress incontinence likely.

Rectocele causes feeling of incomplete defaecation, pain on defaecation, deep dyspareunia.

Diagnosis. Visualisation of bulge and incontinence on coughing.

Treatment. Wait and watch if symptomless. Annual review.

Surgical. Anterior colporrhaphy for cystocele. Diamond shaped excision of epithelium from anterior vaginal wall between urethral orifice and anterior fornix. Edges brought together to form sling supporting neck of bladder and urethra.

Posterior colporrhaphy for rectocele. Triangular shaped excision of epithelium from posterior vaginal wall from perineum to posterior fornix. Edges brought together as for anterior operation.

Combined operations performed. Most common. Manchester repair (Fothergill's operation) in which anterior and posterior colporrhaphy combined with amputation of cervix.

Neoplasm of vagina

All quite rare.

Benign. Cysts occasionally found, e.g. Gartner's (see page 52); implantation cyst following trauma during childbirth or surgery. Epithelial island isolated below healed surface; endometrioma — pocket of endometrium becomes transplanted during curettage. Undergoes typical endometrial changes during menstrual cycle.

Fibroma, lipoma, adenoma occasionally seen.

Treatment. Excision.

Malignant. Primary carcinoma, rare, usually squamous cell (80 per cent). Adenocarcinoma (8 per cent), occasional melanoma.

Recent increase in incidence of clear cell adenocarcinoma of vagina in adolescent girls whose mothers received stilboestrol during early pregnancy, especially before 10th week. Others show higher incidence of adenosis of vagina without progression to malignancy. Stilboestrol quite extensively used in 1950's to 1960's to prevent abortion. Where such history known all girls should be examined annually from age 15.

Adenosis detected by iodine staining of vaginal epithelium,

(Schiller's test), normal epithelial cells stain brown because of glycogen content, other cells lacking glycogen remain white. Other abnormalities may be present in such girls— transverse vaginal epithelial ridges, shortening of anterior fornix, constriction of vagina anterior to cervix, high incidence of adenosis of cervix.

Secondary carcinoma of vagina more common than primary — spread from cervix especially.

Signs and symptoms. May be none. Abnormal cells found on vaginal cytology or ulcer seen on examination. Occasionally, watery or bloody discharge, especially after intercourse.

Inguinal nodes involved in 20 per cent. Pain usually a late symptom.

Investigations. Examination under anaesthesia for biopsy, siting and staging of lesion.

Stage 0. Confined to epithelium
Stage I. Limited to vaginal wall
Stage II. Does not extend to pelvic wall
Stage III. Extends to pelvic wall
Stage IV. Involves bladder or rectum

Treatment. Depends on age, site and stage. Upper vagina carcinoma treated as cervical with attempt to preserve fertility if patient is young and in stage 0 or I. Patient who has enough family or beyond age 50, hysterectomy and vaginectomy.

Stages III and IV radiation alone may be used. Special centres where expertise is concentrated achieve best results.

12. The Uterus

Anatomy

Hollow, pear shaped organ 8 × 5 × 2·5 cm.

Body: upper part, fundus widest between cornuae, i.e. entrances of fallopian tubes, one on each side.

Lower part continuous with cervix at level of internal os. Cervix: lower part. More cylindrical. Projects into anterior wall of vault of vagina.

Structure

Thick muscle layer, myometrium, poorly defined into three sublayers. Fibres arranged in figure-of-eight fashion encircling arterioles so that contraction of fibres compresses vessels thus controlling haemorrhage.

Lining, endometrium, dense stroma supporting columnar epithelium arranged in tubular mucous glands.

Covering, serous membrane, peritoneum closely applied anteriorly and posteriorly. Extended laterally to pelvic walls forming broad ligament. Anterior fold reflects onto bladder to form utero-vesicular pouch. Posterior fold reflects onto rectum to form utero-rectal pouch or pouch of Douglas. Broad ligaments also partially enclose and support ovaries, fallopian tubes, uterine and ovarian arteries, veins, lymphatics, nerves.

Cervix, mainly fibrous tissue, Endocervix of columnar epithelium arranged in branching tubular glands secreting mucin. Lining epithelium gives way abruptly to squamous epithelium of vagina which reflects over cervix to external os.

Internal os lying 2·5 cm inside cavity dermarcates cervix from body.

Ligaments

Uterus held and supported by thickenings of peritoneum and by muscles forming pelvic diaphragm.

Broad ligament extends between lateral wall of pelvis. Round ligaments extend from cornuae antero-inferior to fallopian tubes, through inguinal canals to disperse in labia majora.

Transverse cervical ligaments (cardinal ligaments), main supports, extend from cervix laterally, spreading out fan-like to fascia of pelvic wall.

Pubocervical ligaments extend from cervix to pubis sweeping round base of bladder.

Uterosacral ligaments extend posteriorly on each side of rectum to sacrum.

Development

By 6th week, fetus develops pair of Muellerian ducts extending from body cavity to urogenital sinus. Internal ends become fimbriated ends of fallopian tubes. By 9th week ducts fuse to form a solid cord which canalises to form uterus, cervix and upper 2/3 of vagina. Usually complete by 20th week.

Blood supply. Broad ligament on each side enfolds ovarian artery arising directly from aorta and uterine artery from internal iliac artery. Both vessels run extremely tortuous course sending out numerous branches to fallopian tube, ovary and uterus and uniting at cornua. Tortuous nature allows expansion during pregnancy.

Veins accompany arteries and communicate with ovarian, vesicular, rectal, vaginal, presacral vessels. Join internal iliac veins, inferior vena cava and left renal veins.

Lymphatics. Three complex interconnecting networks within endometrium, myometrium and subperitoneum. Main vessels pass from fundus, body, ovaries, fallopian tubes to para-aortic nodes, from anterior part of body via inguinal canals to superficial inguinal nodes, from cervix via parametrial nodes to internal iliac nodes and to obdurator node. Posterior parts of body send lymphatics via sacral nodes.

Nerves. Uterus receives nerves from sympathetic and parasympathetic systems; sympathetic motor fibres from D5–6, sensory from D10, L1 via presacral and pelvic plexuses; parasympathetic from S2, 3, 4.

Congenital malformations

Development from fusion of two Muellerian ducts may be arrested at any stage.

1. Complete separation with two uteri, two cervices, two vaginae (uterus didelphys)
2. Fusion at vagina but uterus and cervix unfused (uterus bicornis bicollis)
3. One Muellerian duct fails to develop properly and rudimentary horn remains on one side (uterus unicornis)
4. Fusion occurs but septum remains, dividing uterus into two. Usually extends into cervix and may extend into vagina (uterus septus)
5. Fusion occurs but partial septum extends from fundus (uterus subseptus)
6. Fusion occurs but fundus is wide and indented (arcuate uterus)
7. Complete failure of development of Muellerian duct system (absent uterus, cervix, fallopian tubes, upper vagina).

Signs and symptoms. No symptoms until puberty when failure to menstruate leads to discovery of absent uterus. Septate vagina may cause initial coital difficulty. Infertility, abortion, malpresentation, placenta praevia more common. Pregnancy in rudimentary horn may rupture.

Diagnosis. Careful inspection of vagina and cervix. Hysterosalpingography reveals abnormality.

Treatment. Vaginal septum incised. Surgical removal of rudimentary horn if discovered before pregnancy occurs. Where other abnormalities discovered during pregnancy assessment made more frequently especially near term and possible need for Caesarean section kept in mind.

Uterine displacement

Normally adult uterus lies at 90° to plane of vagina, leaning forward over posterior aspect of bladder. In 15 per cent of women uterus is retroverted, i.e. it lies in same plane as vagina or bent back towards sacrum. In childhood uterus is small and normally retroverted.

Types of retroversion are (1) congenital and (2) acquired.

Congenital rarely produces symptoms. Remains mobile. Does not affect pregnancy.

Acquired. Causes: Childbirth, endometriosis, pelvic infection, tumours.

Examination. Bimanual examination reveals, size, shape and position of uterus. If normal size and mobile no special treatment needed. If enlarged and fixed symptoms usually present.

Symptoms. Persistent backache. Dissatisfied defaecation, deep dyspareunia. Dysmenorrhoea.

Treatment. Pessary. Hodge pessary — firm, flattened eliptical — inserted into vagina from posterior fornix to behind symphysis pubis, to retain uterus in anteverted position. Left in position for 6 to 12 weeks. If dyspareunia relieved, surgical correction of retroversion performed.

Operations. Crossen-Gilliam operation in which round ligaments pulled through internal abdominal ring and sutured to back of rectus sheath. Or round ligaments plicated, i.e. shortened by pleating and stitching.

Hysterectomy may be preferred treatment in menopausal women or when no further family wanted and symptoms severe.

Uterine prolapse (displacement)

Definition. Downwards displacement of uterus into vagina.

Cause. Weakness of supporting ligaments and pelvic diaphragm. Almost always history of childbearing. May start soon after parturition but may not appear until well into post-menopause. Contributing factors — increased weight of uterus due to neoplasm, pressure from abdominal contents especially in obesity, straining in constipation. Usually preceded by or accompanying cystocele and rectocele (see page 63).

Stages
1. Cervix below level of ischial spines.
2. Cervix at level of introitus.
3. Procidentia. Fundus at introitus. Vagina everted.

Signs and symptoms. Patient notices lump in vagina. Backache. Frequency and urgency common, due to ready infection of static urine. Stress incontinence common. Unsatisfied defaecation. In 3rd stage, ulceration of cervix with infection and bleeding.

Treatment. Conservative or surgical.

Conservative during fertile years provided adequate control maintained, and when surgery contra-indicated for other reasons.

Surgical. Fothergill's operation if further family required. Vaginal hysterectomy with anterior and posterior colpoperineorrhaphy if no further family wanted.

Conservative treatment involves use of pessaries to maintain uterus in position after manual replacement. Portex solid plastic ring of suitable size inserted. Should cause no discomfort. Left in situ for 12 weeks. Other pessaries used — watch spring; rubber ring with spring embedded; Gelhorn, plastic mushroom keeps position by suction.

Patient instructed to douche with saline daily. Pessary removed and replaced after 12 weeks. Removed if uncomfortable, or causing bleeding.

Endometriosis

Definition. Condition in which tissues identical histologically with endometrium are found in abnormal sites and undergo typical changes throughout menstrual cycle.

Cause. Unknown. Several theories:

1. Retrograde menstruation. Endometrial cells carried backwards through fallopian tubes and embed in ovaries and pouch of Douglas
2. Lymphatic transport
3. Vascular transport
4. Embryonic cell nests activated by hormones

Sites. May be confined to myometrium and then called adenomyosis. Ectopic sites in order of frequency — ovary, pouch of Douglas, broad ligament, sigmoid colon, rectum. Less common sites are bladder, cervix, round ligament, appendix, umbilicus, utero-sacral ligaments.

Pathology. Areas of ectopic endometrium undergo proliferative changes due to oestrogen and progesterone and bleed during menstruation. Blood cannot escape and forms cyst. Serum absorbed leaving thick, tarry residue. Cysts may be any size from pin head to orange. May rupture causing inflammatory reaction with adhesion formation which binds uterus in retroversion and may involve gut and omentum.

Incidence. Rare before 30 years of age. More common among childless women or those who have not conceived for some years.

Signs and symptoms. Symptomless in 25 per cent. Diagnosis made incidentally. In others onset of dysmenorrhoea after years of pain free periods. Menstrual upsets — menorrhagia, polymenorrhoea. Pain usually starts day or two before period, worst during period, diminishes gradually. With large cysts pain may be constant. When gut involved may be painful defaecation. Adhesions and retroversion cause dyspareunia.

Bimanual examination at time of menstruation may reveal tender cysts, in posterior vaginal wall, pouch of Douglas, ovary. Retroverted, fixed, immobile uterus.

Treatment. Surgical removal of cysts, especially large ovarian cysts. Division of adhesions. Restoration of ante-version. Preservation of reproductive function if possible. In older women total hysterectomy may be best.

Hormone treatment cures many cases. Also softens adhesions and reduces cyst sizes preparatory to surgery. Norethisterone acetate, dose rising from 2·5 mg to 15 mg daily in steps of 2·5 mg every 2 weeks. Dose maintained for 9 months. Produces a pseudopregnant state converting endometrium to a pseudodecidua. Amenorrhoea results and cessation of pain causes marked general improvement. Other progestogens and other regimes also successful. Eliminates need for surgery or radiation therapy in many cases especially if diagnosis established early.

Benign tumours of uterus

Fibromyoma (fibroid)

Definition. Tumour of smooth muscle usually arising in myometrium.

Cause. Unknown. Linked to oestrogen production in some way. Growth increases when oestrogen production high, e.g. during pregnancy, atrophy at menopause. Like endometriosis, more common in childless women and in those who last conceived many years ago.

Incidence. Actual incidence not known because often symptomless and remain undiagnosed. May be as high as 30 per cent of women.

Sites. Arise in myometrium and 70 per cent remain in myometrium. Ten per cent grow towards cavity of uterus increasing surface area of endometrium and may become pedunculated. Twenty per cent grow towards peritoneal surface and may become pedunculated.

Size. Most remain small up to 2·5 cm diameter but may grow to 25 lb weight.

Pathology. White colouration with whorled pattern of spindle shaped cells lying within network of fibrous tissue. Pseudocapsule of connective tissue interposed between tumour and normal myometrium which allows shelling out at operation.

Tumour grows very slowly. Blood supply poor and derived from small vessels in pseudocapsule. Tumour may atrophy — the fate of most at menopause — but may degenerate earlier if blood supply or venous drainage impeded. Hyaline degeneration common: areas lose cellular definition and may become cystic. Acute degeneration caused by venous obstruction may occur during pregnancy. Gives rise to signs of 'acute abdomen', condition of red degeneration, so called because of raw beef appearance, due to extravasation of red cells which break down to release haemoglobin.

Rarely malignant change to sarcoma or leiomyosarcoma occurs. Suspected if sudden increase in size.

Volvulus and torsion of pedunculated variety may also cause sudden symptoms and surgical emergency.

Signs and symptoms. Majority are symptomless, others depend on site and size. Submucous, especially pedunculated — menorrhagia, hypermenorrhoea, with clots and pain, occasionally continuous bloody discharge. Subserous may bleed or rupture. Adhesions to gut may cause digestive tract symptoms. Large ones may cause pressure symptoms, e.g. bladder — frequency, dysuria, retention; rectum — constipation, unsatisfied defaecation; lymphatic drainage — ascites.

When present during pregnancy may cause abortion, premature labour, malposition, malpresentation, obstruction, post-partum haemorrhage.

Infertility may be only complaint. Fibromyoma, by distorting uterine cavity make implantation difficult.

Diagnosis. Bimanual examination locates uterus unevenly

enlarged by one or more smooth rounded masses. Uterus usually mobile and masses move with it. Other causes of enlarged uterus must always be excluded, e.g. pregnancy, malignant tumour.

Treatment. Depends on (1) symptoms; (2) age and (3) family status.

1. Observation only. Majority atrophy at menopause
2. Surgical
   (a) myomectomy when infertility is complaint or when further family desired or if submucous pedunculated are easy to remove vaginally
   (b) Hysterectomy if family complete or patient over 40

Carcinoma of cervix

Visible part of cervix projecting into vagina covered with same stratified squamous epithelium as vagina. At or near external os epithelium changes to columnar ciliated variety. Line at which change occurs variable with size of cervix. When a portion of columnar epithelium is visible it shows red against white of surrounding squamous epithelium. Used to be termed an 'erosion' but this term suggests ulceration or, at least, a pathological condition. Better called 'eversion' or 'ectropion'. Transitional region is of particular interest because earliest changes before development of cancer of cervix occur here.

Papanicolaou smear test. Early detection of cytological changes aided by scraping transitional region with wooden spatula and spreading cells thus gathered onto glass slide. Smear fixed with alcohol and stained to show up details of nuclei and cytoplasm. Cell details vary with stage of menstrual cycle, whether oral contraceptives being taken, whether pregnant, whether malignant change is occuring.

Regular smear testing every 2 years regarded as essential to reduce death rate from cervical cancer. When any change detected observations made more frequently and extensively.

Incidence of cervical carcinoma. Two per cent of women develop cervical carcinoma. If it is undiagnosed before becoming clinically obvious, half the number die due to renal failure, infection or secondary spread, no matter what form of treatment adopted. Among women who receive regular routine smear testing, 2 per cent require further investigation but only 0·3 per cent progress to invasive carcinoma.

Age of onset. Majority of non-invasive carcinomas diagnosed by smear test and biopsy occur between 25 and 35. Invasive carcinoma above age 40 with peak about 60.

Types. Ninety-five per cent squamous cell. Four per cent adenocarcinoma. Rare — sarcoma, lymphoma, melanoma.

Cause. Unknown. Wide range of factors implicated. Very rare indeed among virgins. Most common among sexually active women especially when sexual activity started in adolescence. Risk increases with number of sexual partners and with frequency of intercourse. Low incidence among Orthodox Jews who observe law of Niddah which forbids intercourse during menstruation and 7 days after, during pregnancy and post-partum for some months.

Other factors investigated but not proved, e.g. effect of male circumcision, effect of smegma.

Increasing evidence incriminating herpes virus type 2 and spermatazoa. Both carry DNA and by labelling with radioisotope it can be shown to enter cervical epithelial cells while they undergo cell division. Theory is that cells in vicinity of squamo-columnar junction are particularly liable to undergo malignant change when new hormonal balance first established in adolescence. Further vulnerability occurs if an eversion is present and happens to be in an active cellular reproductive phase when a mutagen such as herpes virus or spermatazoa donates DNA to one or more of the reproducing cells.

This establishes a new line of cells which may take years to develop detectable abnormalities and carcinoma.

Premalignant conditions

Metaplasia

Term applied when cell or tissue changes from one type to another. At squamo-columnar junction metaplasia may be first indication of alteration from normal. New cells arise from region of columnar epithelium which do not take up glycogen and do not form normal keratinisation at surface. Such cells do

not stain brown with iodine (Schiller test). Other changes seen
on microscopy increase in number and size and changes in
shape and staining properties of nuclei.

Metaplastic cells may or may not become malignant.

Dysplasia

Similar differences to metaplasia arise in basal cell layer of
squamous epithelium. As new layers of altered cells develop
the old, normal layers above are gradually replaced. New
surface may be white with increased keratosis, do not take up
iodine, appears as islands surrounded by normal epithelium.
Microscopy shows abnormal nuclei with many in mitosis.

Dysplastic cells may or may not become malignant, but a
greater proportion will do so than in metaplastic change.

Carcinoma in situ

Full thickness of epithelium undergoes malignant change
but there has been no penetration through basal membrane
into sub-epithelial layers. Individual cell boundaries indistin-
guishable. No differentiation into layers. Surface either not
keratinised or heavily keratinised. Nuclei densely stained.
Many mitoses throughout epithelium.

Rarely, carcinoma in situ regresses and normal pattern
resumed. Commonly remains unchanged for up to 10 years
then breaks through into sub-epithelium and becomes invasive carcinoma.

Investigations. Biopsy taken when abnormal cells seen on
smear test. May be done while performing colposcopy (see
below) or prior to dilatation and curettage to obtain endometrial samples. Punch biopsy specimens taken from several areas
of cervix especially those failing to take up iodine stain (Schiller test).

Cone biopsy performed to remove cervical canal and margin of normal cervix.

Colposcope is a magnifying, lensed and lighted instrument
enabling a good view of cervix magnified ×6 to ×40. Abnormal areas readily seen after application of 3 per cent acetic
acid, and biopsy more reliable. Areas can be mapped and
photographed for future comparison. Blood vessel pattern
also informative of abnormal sites.

Treatment. Metaplasia and dysplasia subject to colposcopy.

Cone biopsy performed to exclude carcinoma in situ or invasive carcinoma, but if not suspected local areas excised or cauterised. If carcinoma in situ discovered treatment depends on nature of cone biopsied. If whole affected volume has been removed and further family desired, close watch kept on cervix and radical surgery deferred. In all cases of invasive carcinoma, radical surgery with or without radiation necessary to preserve life.

Stages of carcinoma of cervix
0. Carcinoma in situ. Carcinoma entirely intra-epithelial
I. Invasive carcinoma entirely confined to cervix
II. Extension beyond cervix but not to lateral pelvic walls or lower 1/3 vagina
III. Extension to one pelvic wall or lower 1/3 vagina
IV. Spread to bladder, rectum or distant metastases.

Prognosis. Stages 0 and I. Good prognosis with any form of treatment such as conisation, cauterisation or irradiation.

Stage II. Best results with combination of radical surgery and irradiation. Five years survival rate is between 50 and 70 per cent.

Stages III and IV. Radical surgery plus irradiation. Results very poor. Better to avoid extensive surgery and treat palliatively only. Irradiation useful to control haemorrhage, to reduce bone pain or pain from pressure by lymph node enlargement. Analgesia increasing in strength usually needed.

Mainstay of treatment is good nursing care and sympathetic handling.

Endometrial carcinoma
Aetiology. Most commonly arises between 55 and 65 years in single or childless women who have always had profuse or prolonged periods and in whom menopause was delayed beyond 53 years. Other factors commonly associated obesity; hypertension; diabetes mellitus; oestrogen secreting tumour of ovary.

Signs and symptoms. Post-menopausal bleeding always suspicious. Classically, bleeding is slight, watery, irregular, brown, smelly. May be bright, copious. If cervical os obstructed blood banks up, becomes infected, causing general toxic symptoms. Uterus enlarged, tender.

Diagnosis. Dilatation and curettage imperative in all cases of post-menopausal bleeding. Scraping taken serially and kept separate — cervix, then body, then fundus. Adequate curettage reveals carcinoma in 94 per cent of cases.

Other diagnostic measures less reliable. Attempts to establish simple screening measures comparable to Papanicolaou smear for cervical cancer include endocervical aspiration, endometrial smear collecting material by suction, brush, swabs, lavage. Informative results in experienced hands.

Pathology. Eighty per cent adenocarcinoma arising in upper posterior wall of uterus. Slow growth through endometrium. Late spread to myometrium 15 per cent adenoacanthoma. Histologically cells arise from columnar epithelium. Well differentiated cells have better prognosis than poorly differentiated. Anaplastic cells have very poor prognosis. Basis for treatment attempted on grade of carcinoma found and on stage of progress.

Grading
1. Well differentiated
2. Poorly differentiated
3. Anaplastic.

Staging
  0. Dysplasia but no definite evidence of carcinoma
  I. Carcinoma confined to corpus
 II. Extension to cervix
III. Extension beyond uterus but not outside true pelvis
IV. Extension beyond true pelvis or penetrating to mucosa of bladder and rectum.

Treatment. Surgery alone or surgery plus irradiation give best results taking into account stage and grade. Stage I and II with grade 1 differentiation show good survival with simple hysterectomy. Survival progressively worse with stages III and IV and grade 2 and 3.

Irradiation may be by radium or radon implant or by external beam irradiation. May be used alone if surgery contra-indicated or palliatively for inoperable tumour or where lymph node involvement discovered at operation.

Stage III needs radical hysterectomy with prior irradiation and probably post-operative beam irradiation.

Proforma varies at different centres.

Hormone therapy with progesterones halts progress of tumour and metastases. Medroxy-progesterone acetate (Provera) 100 mg, q.i.d. for 6 weeks then b.d. for life.

Spread. Local infiltration to myometrium and beyond into adnexae. Occurs more readily when tumour arises in lower part of uterus. Lymphatic spread occurs late. From lower uterus to iliac nodes then to para-aortic. From upper uterus directly to para-aortic. Blood borne metastases rare but occurs to lungs, adrenals, liver and bones.

Other malignant growths of uterus

Rare. Include leiomyosarcoma (muscle), sarcoma (connective tissue), lymphoma and metastases.

Trophoblastic disease

Definition. Neoplasm following pregnancy. Rare.

Forms

1. Benign. Hydatidiform mole. Abnormal development of placenta. Multiple cyst-like masses of distended villi. Blood vessels scanty or absent
2. Malignant
   a. Invasive mole (Chorio-adenoma destruens). Trophoblastic tissue spreads between cells of myometrium but no destruction of muscle cells
   b. Choriocarcinoma. Trophoblastic tissue invades myometrium with rapid destruction, haemorrhage and early spread to lungs, liver, brain.

Pathology. Trophoblast is foreign to maternal tissues but fails to evoke immunological response. Normally symbiotic relationship exists from about 80th day of pregnancy and invasion of maternal tissue halts. In hydatidiform mole trophoblast takes up fluid and nutrient, swelling into grape like masses with very few blood vessels. In malignant spread trophoblastic tissue continues to penetrate myometrium.

Incidence. One in 6000 pregnancies in European stock rising to 1 in 2000 in Asiatics. Ten per cent of benign moles proceed to become malignant. About 1 in 5000 malignant moles arise after abortion and 1 in 50 000 cases arise after normal pregnancy.

Signs and symptoms. Vaginal bleeding. Persistent morning sickness. Uterus big for length of pregnancy. Hypertension.

Oedema. No fetal parts felt. No fetal movements or heart beat. Urinary chorionic gonadotrophin (HCG) remains elevated.

Bleeding suggests threatened abortion but occurs about 14 to 18 weeks, i.e. several weeks later than usual time for abortion.

Progression to malignant disease suggested by persistent high level of HCG, persistent vaginal bleeding, enlarged uterus, anaemia, weight loss or symptoms arising from metastatic deposits; lungs — dyspnoea, haemoptysis, haemothorax; liver — hepatomegaly, jaundice, altered liver function tests; brain — CVA, headache, coma.

Treatment. Of hydatidiform mole — aid expulsion of mole by digital evacuation. Delay curettage for few days because myometrium thin and vascular.

Of choriocarcinoma — methotrexate 20 mg on two successive days followed by hysterectomy and further methotrexate 20 mg for 3 days. If further family wanted uterus conserved and reliance placed on methotrexate 100 mg daily for 5 day courses with check of serum levels of HCG. Other cytotoxic agents used cyclophosphamide, 6-mercaptopurine, actinomycin-D.

Follow up at monthly interval for 6 months then 3 monthly intervals for 1 year then annually. Pregnancy to be avoided for 1 year at least.

Infections of uterus (endometritis, cervicitis)

Endometritis
Definition. Inflammation of endometrium due to bacterial invasion. May be acute or chronic.

Cause. Gonorrhoea. Streptococcus, Staphylococcus. Tuberculosis. Non-specific.

Endometrium more susceptible to infection following menstruation, abortion, childbirth. Superficial infection unlikely to persist during fertile years because menstruation sheds surface. Chronic infection invades deeper layers and is not cleared out by menstruation.

Gonorrhoea — see page 47.

Signs and symptoms. Streptococcal, staphylococcal, non-specific acute infections.

Menorrhagia; dysmenorrhoea; discharge of purulent material; pelvic pain; low back ache; frequency due to associated trigonitis. General symptoms — pyrexia, malaise.

On examination uterus enlarged. Tender when mobility tested.

Treatment. Antibiotics. Broad spectrum initially while awaiting sensitivity test results. Co-trimoxazole. Amoxicillin. Rest in bed during toxaemic stage. If following abortion, child birth, dilatation and curettage to evacuate retained conception products.

Tubercular endometritis often symptomless and diagnosed during investigations for infertility. D and C performed and curettings examined by expert bacteriologist after Ziehl-Neilsen staining. Other specimens cultured on special media and injected into guinea-pig.

Treatment. Course of antitubercular drugs combination of two of streptomycin, isonicotinic acid hydrazide (IH), para-amino-salicylic acid (PAS), rifampicin and ethambutol. General investigation to reveal source of primary infection, usually in lungs, and examination of close contacts.

13. The Fallopian Tubes (Oviducts)

Anatomy

Right and left thick walled, fine bore tubes 12 cm long extending from uterine cornuae to ovaries.

Structure

Three layers. External peritoneum — part of broad ligament. Middle muscle layer subdivided into outer longitudinal, inner circular fibres. Internal mucous membrane with surface of ciliated columnar cells, much folded and convoluted.

Parts

Medial interstitial portion lies within wall of uterus, 1 to 2 cm. Isthmus 4 cm narrow and fine. Ampulla 6 to 7 cm opens out distally. Terminates in finger-like projections, fimbriae, lying close to ovary. Ampulla is open to peritoneal cavity.

Development

Formed from cranial ends of Mullerian ducts.

Functions

To transport ova from ovary to uterus. Fertilisation takes place in ampulla. Developing zygote moves along tube by peristalsis and action of cilia.

Conditions affecting fallopian tubes

Salpingitis (Greek, *salpigx* — a tube)

Definition. Inflammation of fallopian tubes.

Cause. Spread from neighbouring inflamed organs — appendix, colon, uterus, either directly, most frequently or by lymphatics, e.g. from vagina, or by blood stream, e.g. tuberculosis.

Types. Acute: Streptococcus; staphylococcus; E. coli; Clostridium welchii.

Chronic: Tuberculosis; gonorrhoea.

Terms. Salpingo-oophoritis — combined tubal and ovarian inflammatory disease.

Pyosalpinx — pus retained within tube.

Hydrosalpinx — fluid retained within tube which becomes distended.

Acute salpingitis

Signs and symptoms. Sudden onset lower abdominal pain with pyrexia, toxaemia, purulent discharge, frequency and dysuria. Marked tenderness both iliac fossae and suprapubically. Rigidity and guarding lower abdominal muscles. PV examination usually too painful to continue.

Severe shock may develop very rapidly with Gram-negative infections, especially if spread occurs into peritoneal cavity.

Differential diagnosis. Appendicitis; pyelonephritis; torsion of or haemorrhage from ovarian cyst; ectopic pregnancy.

Treatment. Rest in bed well propped up. Sedate liberally.

Amoxicillin or co-trimoxazole initially while awaiting culture and sensitivity reports. If Gram-negative shock present, i.v. installed and gentamycin, carbenicillin, or cephaloriden given.

Laparotomy may be performed when diagnosis in doubt. Occasionally general peritonitis needs drainage.

Complications. Chronic salpingitis. Infertility.

Chronic salpingitis

May follow acute attack. May be history of gonorrhoea, tuberculosis, puerperal sepsis.

Signs and symptoms. Intermittent low abdominal pain and backache. Vaginal discharge, sometimes foul. Menstrual disturbances. Deep dyspareunia. Infertility.

Occasionally long period of chronic ill health with nothing definite to account for it. Headache, loss of zest, anorexia, weight loss.

On examination tenderness more marked in one iliac fossa. Occasionally mass felt which may be elongated or large and arising out of pelvis. White cell count may show neutrophilia and leucocytosis and ESR usually raised.

Treatment. Surgical — salpingectomy with or without oophorectomy. Drain abscess. Hysterectomy if postmenopausal. Tubercular salpingitis may have no symptoms except infertility. Responds well to antitubercular measures (see page 80). May need salpingotomy to restablish patent tube if further pregnancies desired though results disappointing.

Ectopic pregnancy

Definition. Fertilised ovum implants at site other than endometrium.

Sites. Ninety-nine per cent in fallopian tube. Remainder in ovary or abdominal cavity. Of those implanting in tube, 17 per cent occur in fimbria, 55 per cent in ampulla, 25 per cent in isthmus, 2 per cent in interstitial portion.

Causes. Unknown. Theories: delay in reaching tube with loss of zona pellucida and fertilisation late after ovulation. Distortion of tube by previous salpingitis. Congenital abnormality of tube.

Higher incidence among women using intra-uterine device for contraception.

Termination
1. Tubal abortion 65 per cent
2. Rupture into peritoneal cavity 35 per cent
3. Secondary abdominal pregnancy. Rare.

In tubal abortion conceptus may be absorbed completely; may pass into peritoneal cavity from fimbria and there be absorbed; may remain within tube and become surrounded by blood clot — tubal mole.

In rupture of tube, haemorrhage usually sudden and severe, often before pregnancy suspected, at about time of first missed period. Occasionally, gradual bleeding, or bleeding into broad ligament.

Tubal abortion more common when ectopic in ampulla. Rupture more common from isthmus or interstitial portion.

Signs and symptoms. Amenorrhoea common — one or two missed periods. Lower abdominal pain accompanied by faint at onset. Vaginal bleeding — scanty brown discharge, continues without clots. Usually vague indefinite mass palpable. Occasionally palpation causes rupture of ectopic with sudden massive devastating haemorrhage, severe lower abdominal pain, shock. Later pain and tenderness spreads to epigastrium, with referred shoulder tip pain due to diaphragmatic irritation.

Diagnosis. Not difficult when severe, but subacute cases far from certain. Indicators are falling haemoglobin level, normal white cell count, slight pyrexia, positive pregnancy test, mass palpable, tender fornices especially on movement of cervix. Laparoscopy or culdoscopy may confirm.

Differential diagnosis. Abortion. Ovarian cyst. Pelvic infection. Appendicitis. Ruptured corpus luteum. Salpingitis.

Treatment. Laparotomy. Transfusion, preferably with cross-matched blood. Plasma or rheomacrodex or Group 0 rhesus negative blood, or filtered blood from patient's own peritoneal cavity may be used.

Examination under anaesthesia may precede laparotomy in doubtful cases. Often precipitates rupture hence facilities for immediate laparotomy necessary.

Salpingectomy usually performed as recurrence of ectopics extremely likely if conservative operation attempted.

14. The Ovaries

Anatomy

Paired glands lying against posterior aspect of broad ligament, $4 \times 3 \times 1 \cdot 5$ cm. Attached to broad ligament posteriorly, and to uterus by thickened fold within broad ligament — the ovarian ligament. Posterior surface open to peritoneal cavity. Fallopian tube curves over gland superiorly and fimbriae lie in close proximity.

Structure

Anterior surface lying against broad ligament indented to form hilum at which ovarian artery, venous plexus, lymphatics, sympathetic nerves enter and leave.

Substance divided into wide outer cortex covered with tough fibrous capsule, tunica albuginea, and narrow medullary zone. Cortex composed of Graafian follicles. Each follicle is an endocrine organ and contains a potential ovum. Only about 400 to 500 mature to a ripe ovum in a nomal fertile life span.

Fetal ovary at 20 weeks gestation has 20 million oocytes present. At birth this has reduced to 6 million. By 7 years of age 1/4 to 1/2 million remain. Bulk of Graafian follicles remain dormant as far as maturation of ovum goes but all produce oestrogens until menopause.

Each follicle supported by stromal connective tissue cells which form outer covering — theca externa. Within theca externa lies a further layer derived from stroma, theca interna; these cells produce oestrogens. Third layer, membrana granulosa, composed of columnar cells, lines fluid filled follicle also produces oestrogens and liquor folliculi, fluid filling follicles.

Ripening follicles enlarge up to 1 cm in diameter. Ovum surrounded by liquor folliculi providing nourishment, protection and support. Mature ovum reaches large size, 100 μm, discharged into peritoneal cavity surrounded by (1) zona pel-lucida, thick non-cellular membrane pierced by minute cana-liculi, (2) corona radiata, derived from granulosa cells of theca interna, which continue to nourish ovum in its passage to fallopian tubes.

Follicle space left by departed ovum fills with blood clot and then organises to form corpus luteum. This produces proges-terone for next 2 weeks if fertilisation does not occur and then degenerates to leave fibrous scar, corpus alba. If fertilisation occurs corpus luteum persists into pregnancy.

Other follicles, which do not produce mature ova, degener-ate and leave fibrous scars throughout ovary — atretic follicles.

Blood supply

Arterial blood from (1) ovarian arteries branching directly from aorta, (2) uterine arteries — branches of internal iliac arteries which run a tortuous course within broad ligament and anastamose with ovarian arteries.

Veins — pampiniform plexus unites to form ovarian veins. Right joins inferior vena cava, left joins left renal vein.

Lymphatics accompany arteries to lateral aortic and pre-aortic nodes.

Conditions affecting ovaries

Infection

Always associated with salpingitis (see page 81).

Cysts

Cystic conditions arise frequently in normal structures, e.g. follicles, corpus luteum, rarely endometrial deposits.

Follicle cysts

Most common benign ovarian swelling.

Causes

1. Response to gonadotrophin either natural, or in course of treatment with clomiphene or human placental gonado-trophin or menopausal gonadotrophin in treatment for infertility
2. Thickened tunica albuginea resulting from oophoritis pre-venting rupture of mature follicle

3. In association with Stein-Leventhal syndrome (page 91)
Signs and symptoms. Usually symptomless. Occasionally menorrhagia and dysmenorrhoea. Pain which may simulate appendicitis, cystitis, pyelitis, ectopic pregnancy. Tenderness in lateral fornix. Occasionally lump palpable.

Treatment. Usually regress spontaneously within 3 months. Persistent pain and menorrhagia needs laparotomy and removal of cysts.

Corpus luteum cyst
Usually single cyst which may bleed, causing generalised abdominal pain. May simulate ectopic pregnancy. Often occurs in early normal pregnancy hence pregnancy test positive and differentiation from ectopic difficult.

Occasionally, in normal cycle, corpus luteum fails to involute and secretion of progesterone continues and delays menstruation.

Signs and symptoms. Amenorrhoea or menorrhagia, dysmenorrhoea. Abdominal pain worse in one iliac fossa. Pregnancy test negative (except in instance mentioned above). Tenderness in lateral fornix.

Treatment. Observe. If normal pregnancy present cyst regresses by 12 weeks. Laparotomy if cyst continues to enlarge above 5 cm diameter or still present after 3 months.

Neoplasms

Serous cystadenoma
Definition. Cysts arising from coelomic epithelium, lined with cuboidal cells secreting thin, watery fluid.

Frequency. About 10 per cent of all ovarian tumours.

Age. Rarely occur before 35 years.

Pathology. Slowly grow to 10 cm diameter. Lining cells proliferate to form papillary mass. Occasionally grow outwards. Bilateral in one-third of cases. High proportion become malignant.

Signs and symptoms. Usually none unless complication occurs — haemorrhage, torsion, rupture. Lump felt on bimanual examination.

Treatment. Because of high incidence of malignancy best treatment is oophorectomy but in younger person anxious to have further family cyst only removed. Careful follow up continued for 10 years.

Pseudomucinous cystadenoma

Definition. Cysts arising from coelomic epithelium lined with tall columnar cells secreting mucin which causes tension within the cyst. Diverticular-like outgrowths may become attached daughter cysts.

Frequency. About 12 to 15 per cent of all ovarian tumours.

Age. Thirty to 40 years.

Pathology. May grow rapidly to very large size. Multiloculated. Ingrowth of lining to form papilomata 6 per cent become malignant.

Signs and symptoms. Usually none until lump in lower abdomen noticed. Occasionally complications arise — haemorrhage, torsion, rupture.

Treatment. Oophorectomy in younger age group. Panhysterectomy over 40 years.

Dermoid cysts (benign cystic teratoma)

Definition. Cysts arising from primordial germ cells which may contain structures and elements of any tissue. Most common structures found— teeth, hair, sebaceous material, skin, nails. Occasionally muscle, cartilage, bone, rudiments of gut, glands.

Features. Thick walled: unilocular. Up to 10 to 12 cm diameter. Rarely become malignant.

Incidence. Fifteen to 20 per cent of ovarian tumours.

Age. Twenty to 40 years.

Signs and symptoms. Usually symptomless. Most often discovered on pelvic examination at pregnancy.

Treatment. Ovarian cystectomy in younger age range. Oophorectomy for older patients.

Solid neoplasms

Benign. Fibroma. Brenner tumour.

Malignant. Most common — carcinoma. Rare tumours: granulosa cell tumour. Arrhenoblastoma. Disgerminoma. Embryoma (teratoma). Secondary metastatic carcinoma from stomach (Krukenberg), from uterus (adenocarcinoma).

Fibroma

Definition. Benign tumour composed of bundles of fibrous tissue. Unilateral.

Incidence. About 5 per cent of ovarian tumours.

Age. Over 60 years of age.

Signs and symptoms. Abdominal enlargement due partly to size of tumour — 10 to 20 cm diameter but commonly due to ascites. Occasionally right sided pleural effusion also (Meig's syndrome).

Brenner's tumour

Definition. Similar to fibroma. Histologically different because of presence of epithelial cells in addition to fibrous tissue.

Treatment. Oophorectomy.

Carcinoma of ovary

Primary. May occur at any age but more common in 45 to 55 age group. Usually arise in epithelial tissue of cyctadenoma especially serons cystadenama (page 87). Occasionally pseudomucinous cystadenoma (page 88). Rarely in endometrial deposits.

Signs and symptoms. Usually silent until secondary deposition. Spread may be to contiguous organs: peritoneum; omentum; bowel; fallopian tubes; bladder. Lymphatic spread to para-aortic nodes.

Presence of lump may be noticed early but usually onset of weight loss, anaemia, ascites, first symptoms.

Diagnosis. Cytology of aspirated ascitic fluid. Culdoscopy, laparoscopy or laparotomy.

Treatment. Surgical: pan-hysterectomy, with as complete clearance of suspect tissue as possible including greater omentum.

Radiotherapy: confined to pelvic.

Chemotherapy: cytotoxic agents given locally into peritoneal cavity and orally. Chlorambucil. Thiotepa. Cyclophosphamide.

Prognosis. Poor. Eighty-five per cent mortality within 5 years.

Rare tumours

Granulosa-cell tumour. Produces oestrogen. In young

patients cause precocious puberty, in others menstrual irregularity or post-menopausal bleeding. May become malignant. Metastatic spread to peritoneum, lymph nodes.

Arrhenoblastoma. Produces androgens. De-feminises and later masculinises. May become malignant.

Dysgerminoma. Most commonly arises in true hermaphroditic patient. Malignant.

Malignant teratoma. Occurs in children and young women. Highly malignant, fast growing, metastasises early. Composed of embryonic tissues.

Secondary carcinoma. Fourteen per cent of ovarian malignant tumours. Krukenberg tumour from stomach. Others originate in bowel, breast, colon.

Complications of ovarian tumours

Often precede diagnosis of tumour.

Torsion. May occur intermittently and resolve, or suddenly causing pain, shock, vomiting, sudden enlargement of tumour, tender mass in abdomen. Proceeds to gangrene if untreated.

Treatment. Excision.

Rupture. Rare. Most commonly as result of bimanual examination. Subsequent course depends on type of contents. May resolve completely. May bleed, causing condition similar to ruptured ectopic pregnancy. Pseudomucinous cysts contents may seed throughout peritoneum causing ascites and pseudomyxoma peritonei. Widespread metastases occur from carcinoma.

Infection. Often associated with salpingitis. Causes intermittent pain, pyrexia, tenderness to pressure especially on per vaginam examination. May need urgent surgery.

Haemorrhage. Sudden pain with tense abdominal swelling arising from pelvis. Occasionally amount of blood lost sufficient to cause general symptoms — shock, pallor, air hunger, tachycardia, hypotension.

Incarceration. Fixation of mass in pelvis, usually in pouch of Douglas but can burrow into broad ligament or anteriorly between uterus and bladder. Symptoms, due to pressure on bladder, ureter, blood vessels, lymphatics— frequency, retention, hydronephrosis, venous stasis, swelling of leg, pain.

Treated by removal at laparotomy, though freeing cyst from surrounding structures often difficult and tedious.

Stein-Leventhal syndrome

Definition. Condition in which ovaries become large, cystic, with thickened fibrous outer surface and failure to ovulate.

Cause. Unknown. Possibly enzyme deficiency which causes failure of normal endocrine production. Cysts contain androstenedione and no oestrogen.

Signs and symptoms. Amenorrhoea. Mild virilism with increased growth of hair on face and abdomen, acne, obesity, infertility.

Diagnosis. Pregnanetriol in urine. Laparoscopy.

Treatment. Wedge resection of ovary brings about marked normalisation in 75 per cent cases — onset of ovulation, menstruation, restoration of fertility. Clomiphene or HMG may be used.

15. Pelvic Conditions

Several conditions can affect pelvic soft tissues without involving reproductive organs directly. Cyst of embryological remnants, e.g. of mesonephric tubules and ducts may occur anywhere from ovary to labia. Usually of no significance unless torsion occurs. Cysts of Morgagni — close to ovary. Gartner's cyst of vagina.

Usually diagnosed incidentally on bimanual examination but any lump needs investigation and true nature revealed at laparotomy. Occasionally become very large causing pressure symptoms.

Infections

Acute pelvic cellulitis
   Usually arise following surgery, abortion or childbirth. Common after pelvic irradiation for carcinoma.
   Signs and symptoms. Pyrexia, tachycardia, hypotension, low abdominal pain, tenderness on PV examination.
   Treatment. Immediate high vaginal swab and blood culture to find causative organism and sensitivity. Ampicillin or Amoxicillin given pending results.

Chronic pelvic cellulitis
   Usually history of acute pelvic cellulitis. Thickened, fibrous, broad ligament and adhesions hold uterus rigid.
   Signs and symptoms. Persistent deep ache in pelvis and low back. Dyspareunia. Tenderness on attempting to rock uterus during PV examination.
   Treatment. Highly resistant to antibiotics because of poor blood supply to fibrosed, thickened tissues. Short wave diathermy may give relief. Often hysterectomy resorted to eventually.

Pelvic abscess

Usually a complication arising from other infection, e.g. perforated appendix, diverticulitis, colitis, salpingitis, trauma, etc.

Signs and symptoms. Low abdominal pain. Back pain, mucousy diarrhoea, pyrexia, malaise. Mass in posterior fornix also readily palpable rectally.

Treatment. Incision into pouch of Douglas via posterior fornix (posterior colpotomy) or anterior rectal wall. Antibiotics given. Broad spectrum at first and change to specific according to sensitivity test.

Pelvic peritonitis

Usually secondary to other inflammatory conditions.

Signs and symptoms. Similar to pelvic abscess but uterus remains mobile and no mass felt.

Treatment. Analgesics and antibiotics. Nurse in sitting position to discourage spread to general peritoneum and subphronic abscess.

16. Abortion

Definition

Termination of pregnancy before 28th week either spontaneously or planned.

Spontaneous abortion

Causes. Sixty per cent defective ovum; chromosomal abnormalities, malformation, infection with rubella, syphilis. Fifteen per cent faulty implantation of placenta: placenta praevia, circumvallate placenta. Twenty-five per cent maternal causes: abnormal uterus— retroversion, fibroids, congenital abnormalities, incompetent os — high fever, Rh iso-immunisation, diabetes, thyroid disease, trauma.

Terminology

1. Threatened abortion. Any bleeding during first 28 weeks classified as threatened abortion until proved otherwise
2. Inevitable abortion. Dilatation of os and placental separation make abortion inevitable
3. Complete abortion. Fetus, placenta and decidua completely expelled
4. Incomplete abortion. Some part of secundines still within uterus
5. Missed abortion. Fetus dies and is retained. May be expelled later or may be completely reabsorbed
6. Habitual abortion. Three or more successive pregnancies terminated by spontaneous abortion
7. Therapeutic abortion. Pregnancy terminated before 28 weeks surgically or by drugs when the health of the mother would suffer by its continuation or because of substantial risk that child would suffer such physical or mental abnormality as to be seriously handicapped
8. Criminal abortion. Deliberately induced abortion by any means by any person other than by a qualified doctor for a legal reason as in 7 above.

Differential diagnosis. First trimester bleeding — ectopic pregnancy, mole, cervical polyp, carcinoma, implantation haemorrhage, pyosalpinx, ovarian cyst, metropathia haemorrhagica.

Signs and symptoms. Threatened abortion — bleeding, which may be very heavy. Pain— variable in intensity. Occasionally, no pain. On examination os closed. May settle down to normal pregnancy, may become inevitable or missed abortion.

Inevitable abortion. Bleeding, pain, os open. Fetus already dead. Will proceed to incomplete or complete abortion.

Missed abortion. Fetus dead but not immediately extruded. Signs of pregnancy diminish. Breasts no longer swollen and tender, no morning sickness, uterus shrinks. Pregnancy test negative. End results:

1. Complete absorption of fetus and membranes— common in first 12 weeks
2. Formation of carneous mole — lobulated mass of laminated blood clot due to haemorrhages into choriodecidnal space
3. Macerated fetus— collapsed skull bone, liquified organs
4. Spontaneous expulsion.

Incomplete abortion. Bleeding continues and may be severe. Os open.

Treatment. Threatened abortion— rest in bed under sedation, e.g. promazine (Sparine) 50 mg i.m. t.i.d. or pethidine 100 mg i.m. b.i.d. Cervical inspection to exclude other sources of bleeding. Pregnancy test. If bleeding stops ambulate gradually.

Inevitable abortion— if complete abortion occurs, rest and sedate 24 hours, then D and C. If incomplete, uterus must be emptied before bleeding will stop. Pethidine 100 mg. Operate in theatre under general anaesthetic. Curettage may be manual — finger curettage — or by sponge or ovum forceps. Retained material grasped, forceps turned 90° and withdrawn. Manoeuvre repeated until no further retained products retrieved. Oxytocin 5 units or ergometrine 0·5 mg given i.v. Removed products sent for histological examination to exclude hydatidiform mole or chorioncarcinoma.

Missed abortion — pregnancy obviously not progressing. May be no other signs. Wait 3 weeks. If no sign of spontaneous emptying of uterus abortion induced with i.v. oxytocin. Large amount, up to 100 units per litre, may be needed. Dilatation of os usually succeeds if drip alone fails. Curettage after expulsion of conceptus and membranes.

Habitual abortion — 20 per cent have incompetent os. Abortion from this cause occurs typically between 18th to 24th week. May be prevented by insertion of suture round cervix to keep os closed. Suture left in situ until danger of abortion or premature labour over. Removed at 37 weeks or Caesarean section performed.

Other causes of habitual abortion sought — anaemia, uterine abnormalities, fibroids — corrected, if possible, between pregnancies.

Legal and criminal abortion

English Abortion Act of 1967 gives clear guidance for legal abortion in United Kingdom. Two practitioners must agree that continuation would be detrimental to physical or mental health of mother, or any existing children of her family, or there is substantial risk that child would suffer from mental or physical abnormality to a degree suffcient to cause serious handicap. Operation must be performed in registered premises and notified to Chief Medical Officer of Ministry of Health.

In Australia, law less specific, but abortion performed when mother's life at risk by continuation. Common reasons — hypertension, chronic nephritis, cardiac disease, rubella in first trimester, psychiatric reasons. Any doctor can perform operation if he conscientiously believes it to be necessary. Need not be in special hospital and notification not required. However, doctors advised to seek second opinion, especially if grounds are psychological, and to operate only in reputable premises.

Abortion performed by person other than qualified medical practitioner, or by a doctor purely for social reasons, is illegal.

In some countries no reason is needed to abort, but in all it must be carried out by medical practitioner. In other countries all induced abortions are illegal.

Methods
First trimester. 1. Dilatation and curettage. Carried out in proper theatre under general anaesthetic. Cervix dilated with Hegar's dilators to size 12. Conceptus removed with sponge holding forceps using twisting action to ensure no damage to uterus. Gentle curettage follows then digital examination. Ergometrine 0·5 mg given i.m. and cervix observed for bleeding.

2. Suction. Tubes up to 14 mm diameter with side hole inserted through dilated cervix. Suction at 600 g/cm^2 applied via ordinary theatre suction apparatus.

Second trimester. 1. Hysterectomy similar to Caesarean section.

2. Intra-amniotic injection of hypertonic saline.

3. Intra-amniotic infusion of prostaglandins.

In third trimester term 'abortion' not used, instead, 'induction of labour'. Object usually to produce living baby under circumstances where continuation of pregnancy would be dangerous to mother, child or both.

Dangers of induced abortion
1. Sepsis. Common after criminal abortion. Rare with proper facilities, precautions and antibiotics
2. Perforation of uterus into peritoneal cavity, bladder, rectum
3. Embolism, from forcible lavage
4. Red cell haemolysis, from lavage solution being forced into circulation, leading to haemoglobinaemia and acute renal failure
5. Haemorrhage.

Septic abortion

Definition. Infection of uterus following abortion.
Incidence. Varies in different parts of world. Highest in primitive countries and where legal abortion is denied.
Organisms. 80 per cent endogenous anaerobic. Streptococci, staphylococci, E. coli, confined to endometrium.

Fifteen per cent spread to myometrium, adnexae or systemic, Chlostridia and Gram-negative organisms.

Signs and symptoms. Pyrexia, tachycardia, offensive vaginal discharge. Tenderness over uterus and fornices. Leukocytosis over 15 000 per mm^3.

Investigation. Vaginal swab for immediate smear examination, culture and sensitivity. Blood cultures. Urea, electrolytes, blood gases, pH, fibrinogen studies.

Treatment. Pending sensitivity results, ampicillin or amoxicillin 1 g 6 hourly i.v. and streptomycin 0·5 g i.m. twice daily. If gas gangrene suspected give anti gas gangrene serum.

D and C if bleeding persists. Transfusion if necessary.

Gram-negative septicaemia — severe form of post-partum or post-abortal infection caused by endogenous organisms especially E. coli. High mortality. Intense vasoconstriction of venules preventing adequate venous return. Thrombosis of hepatic, pulmonary and renal vessels. Low cardiac output.

Diagnosis. Low BP, low CVP in spite of adequate fluid replacement. Pyrexia. Leucocytosis. Occasionally leucopenia — grave sign.

Treatment. Blood and fluid replacement. High doses of antibiotics, e.g. benzyl penicillin 30 million units daily i.m., ampicillin or amoxicillin 4 g daily i.v. Gentamycin, cephalosporin or other antibiotic known to be effective against Gram-negative organisms used pending sensitivity results.

Acidosis corrected by i.v. sodium bicarbonate. Chlorpromazine 50 mg 6 hourly reduces shock. Corticosteroids, e.g. Solucortef 500 mg/day for one week, increases cellular permeability. Isoprenalin drip 1 μg/minute dilates peripheral vessels.

17. The Breast

Development

Downgrowths of ectoderm occur at 16 weeks gestation. Fifteen to 20 branches develop spreading into mesenchyme. Later become lobes. Distal ends become alveoli. Canalisation of these hitherto solid cords occurs at 32 weeks. Mesenchyme proliferates at surface at 40 weeks and points outward to form nipple.

Two or 3 years before menarche further development starts as oestrogen levels increase. Duct system proliferates to form lobes. Initially, major development lies immediately below areolar raising breast buds. Later increased fat deposition round duct system causes major increase in breast size. After onset of ovulation, progesterone also influences development, mainly increasing acini.

During pregnancy areolar become darker, duct system and acini become active, nipples become bigger, sebaceous glands become prominent — Montgomery's tubercles — providing sebum to keep nipple supple and pliant.

Structure

Fifteen to 20 lobes separated by fibrous septa. Each lobular duct dilates within nipple to form lactiferous sinus which opens onto surface. Each lobe subdivided into lobules composed of acini arranged round central duct. Much fat lies among and surrounding acini, ducts, lobules and lobes.

Size

Usually one breast larger than other. Great variation in size and shape. Usually hemispherical overlying pectoralis major muscle from 2nd to 5th rib with tail extending into axilla.

Vessels

Blood supplied by rich arterial network derived from axillary, internal mammary and intercostal arteries.

Venous drainage passes from circulus venosus surrounding base of nipple, radially to axillary and mammary veins.

Lymphatics originate in walls of lactiferous ducts and in the skin and subcutaneous tissue. Form sub-areolar plexus and pass radially to join those of pectoralis major. Lateral and superior parts drain to axillary glands. Medial part drains to internal mammary nodes. Few lymph channels unite with those of opposite breast. Few pass inferiorly to rectus abdominis sheath and thence to liver.

Nerves

Derived from anterior and lateral cutaneous branches of 4th, 5th, 6th thoracic nerves.

Cyclic changes

Breast sensitive to cyclic hormonal changes. Oestrogen causes ductal activity and increases membrane permeability, progesterone increased acinal activity. Maximum effect 3 to 4 days before menstruation resulting in fullness of breasts, occasionally tenderness.

Changes during pregnancy

Increasing fullness of breasts and hypersensitivity occurs week to 10 days after first missed period. May be first indication of pregnancy. Venous dilatation shows blue network at 8 weeks. Nipple enlargement, darkening of areolar, growth of areolar sebaceous gland, Montgomery's tubercles by 12 weeks. At 28 weeks thin watery fluid may be expressed.

Oestrogen suppresses prolactin production. Childbirth removes source of extra oestrogen and prolactin then influences acini to start milk production. Suckling stimulates oxytocin production and milk ejection starts under its influence.

Breast examination

Regular self examination recommended for the early detection of new breast lumps. All breasts contain lumps which are normal structures. Many women complain that they cannot distinguish normal from abnormal lumps. Normal lumps are smooth, rounded, rarely larger than 1 cm in diameter, non-tender, mobile, almost always corresponding normal lumps found bilaterally. Abnormal lumps usually unilateral, may be tender, grow to be larger than 1 cm; may be hard, fixed, irregular in outline.

Self examination should be systematic, regular and complete not merely a quick palpation when falling asleep only when remembered. Woman should stand or sit before mirror with arm to sides. Careful inspection of shape, contour, size of each breast, position and state of nipple and areolar. Arms then raised above head and same observations made. In particular, any irregularity of normal smooth contour noted, dimpling of skin, nipple retraction or tightness of skin. Then, while lying flat breast divided into four quadrants. Each quadrant systematically palpated, using pads of fingers, starting from nipple and working to periphery. Fingers placed on skin and skin moved circularly against underlying structures. Right hand used to palpate left breast and left hand for right breast. If suspicious lump located woman should see own doctor.

If he agrees that lump is suspicious mammography may be ordered. He will also feel for associated axillary and supraclavicular nodes which cannot be done satisfactorily by self examination.

Conditions affecting breasts

Absent breast development
May be due to ovarian agenesis, ovarian atrophy or local factors. If menarche fails to occur oestrogen levels determined. If deficient, oestrogens will cause breast development.

Small breasts
In menstruating woman not improved with oestrogen. Cosmetic surgery, e.g. silastic implant, gives pleasing result especially if small size is an embarrassment or cause of psychological upset.

Large breasts
Disproportionately large breasts amenable to plastic surgery usually with satisfactory psychological results.

Inverted nipples
Congenital deformity of no consequence unless continuing into pregnancy and afterwards preventing breast feeding. May

be corrected by manipulation especially during pregnancy and by wearing nipple shield.

Inversion of previously normal nipple suspicious of underlying pathology and needs investigation.

Gynaecomastia

Definition. Abnormal breast development in the male.

Causes. Slight degree of gynaecomastia at puberty which usually regresses.

Marked development at any age indicates excess oestrogen either endogenous from tumour or exogenous, e.g. in treatment of prostatic carcinoma with stilboestrol or self administered by female impersonators or for psychiatric reasons.

Investigations. Urinary 17-ketosteroids measured, also response to ACTH (no increase suggests independent tumour), and response to steroids (no decrease similar).

Treatment. Removal of source of oestrogen. Breast usually regresses. Occasionally mastectomy required especially in young sensitive men.

Infections

Most common in first 2 months post-partum. Usual organisms — staphylococci, streptococci.

Pathology. Infection via cracked nipple. Abscess occupies lobe. Rarely spreads to neighbouring lobes.

Treatment. Antibiotic according to sensitivity test. Rarely needs incision and drainage.

Mammary duct ectasia

Definition. Inflammatory condition of ducts in and just below nipple. Ducts become filled with cellular debris and lipid containing material.

Cause. Unknown.

Age. Older women near menopause.

Signs and symptoms. Intermittent pain and local inflammation. Occasionally discharge which may be bloody. Nipple retraction.

Treatment. Exploration and biopsy to exclude carcinoma. Excision of affected lobe.

Benign tumours

1. Fibroadenoma

2. Duct papilloma
3. Mesenchymal (not peculiar to breast) lipoma, angioma, fibroma.

1. Fibroadenoma

Definition. Compound mass of fibrous and glandular hyperplasia in varying proportion.

Age. Under 30 years.

Signs and symptoms. Firm, lobulated, smooth, easily moveable lump usually less than 2 cm in diameter.

Treatment. Removal of lump for cytology to exclude carcinoma.

2. Duct papilloma

Definition. Mass caused by epithelial hyperplasia within lactiferous duct commonly close to nipple.

Age. Fifty to 60 years.

Signs and symptoms. Discharge from nipple often blood stained. Mass usually quite small and difficult to palpate. Pressure over location causes increased discharge. Rarely painful.

Treatment. Exploration and removal for cytology to exclude carcinoma.

3. Mesenchymal tumours

May arise in breast tissue as likely as anywhere else. Usually small, smooth, mobile. Should be removed to exclude carcinoma.

Fibrocystic mazoplasia

Definition. Exaggeration of normal cyclical changes occuring in ductal and acinar tissues in response to oestrogen and progesterone stimulation. May be diffuse affecting both breasts or localised to one gland or one lobe within a gland.

Age. Reproductive years. More common in childless women.

Signs and symptoms. Very variable. Breast fullness and tenderness before menstruation. Increasing nodularity and ropiness with cyst formation. (Blue-domed cysts of Blood-good — so named because of their appearance on section.)

Treatment. Full explanation and discussion. Reassurance that condition is not pre-cancerous. Diuretic daily for 7 to 10 days pre-menstrually. When condition confined to one lobe with one or two larger cysts, aspiration of fluid from cyst causes complete disappearance of lump.

Malignant tumours

Breast carcinoma most common malignant tumour in females.

Age. Biphasic incidence. Steady increase between 20 and 50 then reduction and second peak at 65.

Other factors. Some basis for hereditary susceptibility. More common in childless women. Grow more rapidly under influence of oestrogen, e.g. during pregnancy or with oestrogen therapy.

Environmental factors play unknown part. Less common in oriental women, those who breast feed, thin women. More common in those with some hormonal dysfunction — thyroid atrophy, ovarian stromal hyperplasia, some pituitary tumours — and in those who have had carcinoma in opposite breast.

Site of tumour. Sixty per cent upper lateral quadrant. Almost always arise in duct epithelium and penetrate through basement membrane to invade stroma.

Signs and symptoms. Most often patient notices lump herself. Usually painless. Occasionally nipple discharge, inversion of nipple, eczema of nipple. Sometimes disease advanced when diagnosed with ulcer formation or secondary spread to bones (pathological fracture, bone pain), lung (cough, haemophysis) liver (jaundice).

Investigation. Full history and physical examination. Cytology studies of nipple discharge. Mammography, thermography. Aspiration of cyst fluid and cytology studies. Biopsy with frozen section.

Assessment. Clinical staging and pathological grading.
Stages:
1. Localised growth or Paget's disease of nipple or nipple retraction
2. Plus mobile axillary nodes
3. Immobile tumour attached to pectoralis muscle or to skin or fixed axillary nodes or supraclavicular nodes
4. Distant metastases.
T.N.M. Classification becoming widely used.

T: Tumour
N: Nodes
M: Metastases

Number indicating severity allocated to each letter, e.g. tumour of 4 cm with mobile axillary node and no metastases would be T2, N1, M0:

T1: Up to 2 cm diameter
T2: 2–5 cm
T3: 5–10 cm
T4: over 10 cm
N0: No nodes
N1: Mobile axillary nodes
N2: Fixed axillary nodes
N3: Palpable supraclavicular nodes
M0: No distant metastases
M1: Metastases present.

Grading of tumour. Determined by histological appearance of biopsy.

Grade I. Well differentiated cells. Recognisable columnar cells arranged in tubules in fibrous stroma.

Grade II. Less well differentiated. Spheroidal cells in cords and clumps with attempted tubule formation.

Grade III. Undifferentiated polygonal cells. Rapidly progressive with early metastases.

Treatment. Surgery. Radiation. Cytotoxic drugs. Depends very much on staging and grading. Stage 1, Grade 1, offers best hope with 80 to 90 per cent 5 year survival. Stage 3. Five to 10 per cent, 5 year survival. Stage 4. Death within 1 year.

Stage 2 with Grade II or III tumours present problems of how vigorously to treat. Extensive deforming surgery with little chance of success may be considered unwarranted.

Operations 1. *Radical mastectomy* (Halsted Operation) Standard for lateral hemisphere growths of Stage 1 or 2. Breast, pectoralis muscles and axillary nodes removed.

2. *Modified radical mastectomy* (Patey operation). Pectoralis major muscle retained.

3. *Extended radical mastectomy* (Urban operation). Lateral portion of sternum, second to fifth costal cartilages, internal mammary nodes and nearby parietal pleura removed. Specially useful for medial hemisphere tumours.

Radiotherapy. Doubtful if any benefit to Stage 1 carcinoma. In fact, patients who have only mastectomy, have better record of survival than those who also have radiotherapy.

At present radiotherapy best reserved for limited application to affected nodes and for relief of bone pain from metastases.

Cytotoxic drugs. Local, wound irrigation to kill off 'spilled' malignant cells.

General, Thiotepa 2 mg/kg/i.v. for 3 days post-operatively may reduce spread of metastases resulting from operative manipulation.

Paget's disease of nipple

Definition. Red, scaly, eczematous lesion of nipple associated with carcinoma of breast.

Pathology. Histology reveals multiple clear cells with a halo appearance round abnormal nuclei — Paget's cells. Underlying carcinoma may not be palpable. Usually arises within main duct and extending to skin of nipple.

Treatment. Early mastectomy gives excellent result but often diagnosis not made until axillary nodes involved.

18. Gynaecological Procedures

General considerations

Gynaecology is a highly specialised field dealing with those parts of the body many people have difficulty and embarrassment talking about. Anticipation of investigation and treatment may be so distasteful to the patient that she will delay seeking advice and help until it is imperative and even then she may be too shy to give a full history. In the most extreme case there are some cultures in which a husband will let his wife die rather than allow her to undergo an examination by a male doctor. Fortunately such cases are rare but in societies where immigrant populations are present it is as well to be aware of the possibility.

Nursing gynaecological cases requires the development of special skills in interpersonal relationships if the sensitivities of the patient are not to be offended; and if the threat, real or imagined, to a woman's femininity is to be minimised. Most women welcome an opportunity to discuss sexual matters with another woman and will reveal their worries more readily to a sympathetic nurse than to a doctor. It is essential for nurses in gynaecology to be well informed, knowledgeable, sensitive and sympathetic.

Gynaecological examination

Nurses duties to inform patient and allay fears, to stay with patient and comfort her, to see that doctor has everything necessary, to assist when needed, to reassure and make patient comfortable afterwards.

After general and abdominal examination, vaginal examination performed. Nurse helps place patient in required position — usually dorsal but occasionally lateral or Sims (see below).

Requirements for vaginal examination
  Tray or trolley containing:

> 2 kidney dishes: 1 for swabs and gauze, 1 for used instruments
> 2 lotion bowls: 1 for antiseptic lotion, 1 for lubricant
> Instruments: speculae, sponge holders, vulsellum, tenaculum, sounds
> Others: gloves, gown
> Often swabs and smears taken
> Requirements: slide, spatulae, swabs on sticks, alcohol fixative, pencil, laboratory slips.

Gynaecological positions
1. Dorsal. Flat on back with knees drawn up and thighs apart. Arms to sides and head relaxed to prevent tension in abdominal muscles. Most useful for bivalve speculum and bimanual examination
2. Lateral. Lying on left side with hips and knees flexed and buttocks to edge of bed. Most useful for introduction of Sim's speculum
3. Sim's position. Lying on side, usually left, with left arm behind, left leg flexed to 30° at hip and knee, right hip and knee flexed to 90°
4. Lithotomy position. Flat on back with legs supported in stirrups and buttocks brought to edge of divided mattress. Most commonly used while patient anaesthetised for more detailed bimanual examination, operations via vagina, D and C, etc.
5. Knee-chest position (genu-pectoral). Patient kneels on table with head cradled on folded arms and buttocks raised. Allows ready access to posterior fornix, causes abdominal viscera to fall away from pelvis removing them from possibility of injury during colpotomy and culdoscopy.

Papanicolaou smear
  With clear view of cervix scraping taken from margin of cervical os using spatula. (Recent claims made for better specimens if plastic spatula used rather than wood. Wood surface tends to absorb and retain cells.)

Second specimen taken from within os using cotton wool swab rotated gently inside os.

Third specimen taken from vaginal vault posterior fornix.

All three specimens spread on one clean glass slide. Fixed with 95 per cent alcohol, labelled and sent to laboratory when dry. Request form should state date of last period, whether pregnant or not, whether on oral contraception, clinical appearance of vagina and cervix.

Cervical smears for cytology taken before any other examination has disturbed surface cells.

Endometrial biopsy

To obtain specimen of endometrium without resorting to general anaesthetic and dilatation of os.

Novak's curette introduced into uterine cavity to collect small specimen. Best obtained before expected period when endometrium will show cells in secretory phase if ovulation and progesterone secretion normal.

Colposcopy

Patient placed in lithotomy position and table tilted so that she is reclining at 45°. Colposcope inserted to obtain magnified view of cervix. Magnification variable ×6 to ×40. Monitor attachments allow extra eye-pieces to enable students to view simultaneously. Also camera for permanent recording.

Cervix painted with 3 per cent acetic acid or iodine to show up abnormal areas. Biopsy specimens taken from suspected areas. Diathermy may be applied.

Procedure is painless but patient may need lots of reassurance and comfort especially if investigation lengthy.

Tubal insufflation (Rubin's test)

Carbon dioxide under pressure blown through uterus and fallopian tubes via cannula in cervix. Cannula must be tight fitting to prevent leaks. Pressure up to 200 mm Hg exerted and machine switched off. If pressure is maintained both tubes are blocked. If steady fall occurs at least one tube patent. Stethoscope over iliac fossa may detect hiss of escaping gas.

Simple diagnostic test. May also clear away minor blocks.

Patient usually in lithotomy position. Sedative may be given 1/2 hour beforehand.

Hysterosalpingography

Radio-opaque substance inserted into uterine cavity and fallopian tubes via cannula in cervix. Outlines cavity and tubes and escape into peritoneal cavity denotes patentcy of one or both tubes. More informative than Rubin's test.

No special pre-operative care needed apart from mild sedative.

Gynaegram

Air introduced into peritoneal cavity via needle through abdominal wall. This provides a contrast medium for X-rays, and outlines abdominal organs. When patient in Trendelenberg position air occupies pelvis and abnormalities of uterus, tubes, ovaries show up.

Procedure done without anaesthesia. No pain or discomfort experienced. Amount of air injected quickly absorbed. Bladder and rectum must be empty.

Gynaecological operations — minor

Dilatation and currettage

Cervix dilated gradually with Hegar's dilators and endometrium scraped away with curettes. Ideally amount of endometrium remaining will resemble that following normal menstruation.

Indications

1. Diagnostic. To establish cause of abnormal bleeding in hypermenorrhoea, menorrhagia, post-menopausal bleeding. To ensure absence or presence of carcinoma.
2. Therapeutic. To evacuate uterus completely in incomplete abortion, mole, polyp, missed abortion, retained placental products. To correct dysfunctional menorrhagia and dysmenorrhoea. To terminate pregnancy.

Complications. Haemorrhage. Infection. Perforation. Cervical tear.

Preparation. Explanation often needed that curettage does not sterilise people. Avoid use of word 'scrape'. Restrict intake for 8 hours. Premedication should include atropine to prevent 'cervical shock' — rare complication arising when cervix dilated causing severe hypotension, circulatory failure, cardiac arrest.

Empty bladder and rectum.

Operation. After anaesthesia patient placed in lithotomy position. Perineum, vulva and vagina prepared with aqueous chlorhexidine. Catheter passed to ensure empty bladder. Drapes applied. Adequate view obtained with Auvard or similar speculum. Anterior lip of cervix grasped with volsellum forceps. Length and direction of uterine cavity determined with uterine sound.

Cervix dilated with successive Hegar's dilators. Curette introduced and systematically applied to ensure surface completely treated. Finger introduced finally to ensure no remnants left.

Specimens put up in formalin 10 per cent and sent for histology.

Pad applied and legs lowered carefully.

Post-operative care. While anaesthetised general observation of colour, pulse, blood pressure, state of airway taken and recorded. Patient kept flat until conscious. Vaginal loss monitored. Usually patient ambulatory 4 to 6 hours after D and C depending on reason for its performance.

Management of complications

Haemorrhage. Indicates incomplete emptying of uterus, or relaxation of uterine tone or cervical damage.

Ergometrine 0·5 mg i.m. and external uterine massage will contract uterus. If bleeding continues speculum examination required. May be necessary to repeat curettage. Uterine packs rarely required and should be removed within 24 hours if used.

Infection. High vaginal swab taken for culture and sensitivity. Co-trimoxazole, amoxicillin, Kanamycin may be used pending sensitivity results.

Perforation. Anti-infective measures instituted. Small hole heals without need for further intervention. Observations for peritonitis, paralytic ileus, haemorrhage carried out meticulously.

Large holes will need laparotomy and careful inspection of bowel which may have been damaged. Usually hole in uterus oversewn and heals well. Occasionally hysterectomy required.

Laceration of cervix. Occasionally ligation of bleeding vessel needed.

Insertion of intra-uterine device (IUD)

Usually done as office procedure soon after menstruation without anaesthetic. Occasionally, if there has never been a pregnancy, general anaesthesia employed. If so, should be done in hospital and all pre-anaesthetic precautions taken. Otherwise, only emptying of bladder required.

Patient placed in dorsal position and good view of cervix obtained. Anterior lip grasped with vulsellum forceps. Size and direction of cavity sounded. Device inserted according to makers instructions. Most now have tell-tale nylon monofilament thread left extending through os into vagina. Most are radio-opaque. Both characteristics aid in ensuring that device is properly in situ or locating it when 'lost'.

Complications. Occasionally patient suffers low abdominal cramps after insertion. Usually settles within hour or 2. May need mild analgesia. Rarely: hypotension, pallor, nausea, rapid pulse when device passed through cervix. Prevented by injecting atropine 0·6 mg, 30 minutes before procedure.

Usually patient not inconvenienced. Instructed to insert finger after menstruation and locate threads. To return 1 month after insertion for check-up, and to return at once if in doubt.

Sometimes periods prolonged and heavy with IUD. More likely to occur if device poorly positioned or too small or too large. Best removed and re-inserted after next period.

High incidence of ectopic pregnancy with IUD. Patient should be warned to attend if period missed.

Major surgery

Hysterectomy

Removal of uterus. Type of operation depends on reason for performing it.

Total hysterectomy implies removal of body and cervix.

Subtotal hysterectomy — body only.

Wertheim's hysterectomy consists of total hysterectomy at least upper third of vagina, broad ligaments including parametrium, cardinal ligaments, uterosacral ligaments, both tubes and ovaries and all pelvic lymph nodes. Usually performed for carcinoma of body of uterus or of cervix.

Vaginal hysterectomy means total hysterectomy carried out via the vagina. Performed for prolapse provided uterus not grossly enlarged or distorted with fibroids or has been subjected to previous abdominal surgery or suffered inflammatory processes.

Pre-operative preparation. Patient admitted several days pre-operatively to familiarise her with staff and to provide opportunity for her to ask questions and relieve anxiety. Breathing and leg exercises started. Skin prepared with bath and shave. Bowels emptied by enema evening before.

If prolapse severe and procidentia present local treatment with glycerine and acriflavine packs may be required before operation. Repeated b.d. and patient remains in bed wearing pad and T binder.

Post-operative management. Patient nursed with one or two pillows for 24 hours and then assumes a sitting position gradually.

Observations of colour, pulse, blood pressure, mental state, vaginal loss, urinary output recorded every 15 minutes initially. Longer intervals as progress maintained.

Analgesics given liberally for first 24 hours. Later on analgesics given half hour before procedures which may cause pain, e.g. coughing exercises, physiotherapy. This makes procedure less feared and therefore more effective.

Perineal toilet carried out 4 hourly. Vaginal pack removed at 24 hours.

Urinary output monitored and catheter passed at 24 hours if normal micturition has not occured by that time. If catheter in situ, free drainage for 4 days then intermittently released 4 hourly to regain bladder tone. Catheter removed on 6th day, or before that if passing urine round catheter. Retention of residual urine of more than 60 ml avoided by twice daily catheterization.

While indwelling catheter present Neomycin instilled t.i.d. and retained for 15 minutes each time.

Bowel actions stimulated with aperient on second night followed by enema or suppository following morning. Distension with gas treated by passing flatus tube and with charcoal tablets.

Usually early ambulation encouraged, sitting out on 1st

day, walking to toilet on second day with assistance. Legs exercised frequently to maintain muscle pump.

Discharged home about 10 days and follow-up appointment made for 6 weeks.

Wertheim's hysterectomy — special care

Performed, usually, for carcinoma of cervix or body. Patient admitted and investigated to exclude metastases or ureteric involvement— chest X-ray, IVP. Blood collected for grouping and cross matching.

Preliminary examination performed under anaesthesia. D and C carried out. Biopsy of cervix.

Some centres irradiate uterine cavity with radon at this stage and hysterectomy carried out 6 weeks later. Others proceed at once to hysterectomy without irradiation.

Post-operative care. I.v. fluids continued until danger of paralytic ileus over.

Drain tube in abdominal wound dressing within 24 hours and then as required until drainage minimal and removed. Vaginal T-drain tube connected to underwater seal. Amount of drainage recorded.

Usually kept in situ until drainage minimal then removed. Suture line exposed on 7th day and betadine lotion applied. Sutures removed 10 to 14 days.

Urine output recorded and intermittent release of catheter instituted early to reduce risk of bladder atony.

Early ambulation encouraged to reduce risk of DVT.

Ruptured ectopic pregnancy

Surgical emergency. Often arises before patient is aware of pregnancy.

Patient admitted in state of shock having fainted and complained of abdominal pain in iliac fossa. Frequently shoulder tip pain present.

I.v. drip installed. Blood collected for grouping and cross matching. Drip started with Group 0 Rh-negative blood and changed as soon as matched blood available. Patients own blood can be collected from peritoneum, filtered and returned i.v.

Operating theatre alerted. Patient receives very little preparation apart from restricting oral fluids. Skin preparation can be performed when anaesthetised.

Anaesthetisation may present problems if food or fluid has been ingested lately. Risk diminished by applying cricoid pressure as soon as patient asleep until endotracheal tube inserted. Then stomach tube can be installed safely.

Post-operative recovery is usually swift and uneventful.

Tubal ligation

Frequent method of contraception. Patient should be warned of irreversible nature of operation. (Though microsurgical techniques for end-to-end anastomosis proving successful.) Many centres require husband's signature that operation is being done with his knowledge.

No special preparation required. Post-operative course usually rapid and uneventful.

Operations for prolapse

Anterior colporrhaphy — to tighten bladder support and restore urethral angle to prevent stress incontinence.

Posterior colporrhaphy — to restore support to rectal wall.

Manchester repair (Fothergill's operation) — combination of anterior and posterior colporrhaphy plus amputation of cervix.

Pre-operative care. Difficulty persuading women to consult gynaecologist for correction of symptoms which are not causing pain, bleeding or ill health. Many women expect to suffer conditions after childbearing and tolerate surprising degrees of inconvenience unnecessarily.

Few days in hospital resting in bed improves feeling of well being and reduces pelvic congestion.

Bowels emptied with aperient and simple enema.

Operation. Triangular areas of vaginal epithelium removed anteriorly and posteriorly. Cervix amputated — cardinal ligaments shortened by incision, ligation and resuturing to cervical stump. This pulls cervical stump posteriorly and levers uterus to anteverted position. Posteriorly levatores ani muscles brought together in midline to support anterior rectal wall. Edges of vaginal epithelial incisions brought together in midline anteriorly and posteriorly and sutured. Vagina packed with vaseline gauze.

Post-operative care. Patient nursed flat until conscious then nursed in position of greatest comfort.

Pack removed after 24 hours. Subsequent care depends on

surgeons preference, some like patient to have sitz baths, others vaginal douches, others heat lamp and antiseptic spray.

If catheter in situ free drainage allowed for 3 to 5 days then intermittent release of clamp to encourage regain of bladder tone. If no catheter installed at operation careful observation made to ensure distension does not occur. If no urine passed for 8 hours catheter inserted and repeated twice daily to ensure residual urine of not more than 60 ml.

Bowels encouraged to open without straining. Faeces kept soft with daily agarol and bulk provided with high fibre diet. Fluids given liberally as soon as tolerated.

Early ambulation encouraged from first post-operative day. Patient discharged when healing satisfactory usually about 10th day and appointment made for 6 week check-up.

Repair of complete tear involves refashioning posterior vaginal wall and anterior rectal wall and rejoining severed anal sphincter. While healing taking place bowels confined with low residue diet, tincture of opium or lomotil for 7 days. Then rectal contents softened with oil enema and liquid paraffin orally.

Vulvectomy

Extensive excision of skin from area bounded by anterior superior iliac spines superiorly, lesser trochanters inferiorly and from anal margin to symphysis pubis, including labia minora and clitoris but leaving urethral orifice intact. Inguinal nodes also removed.

Pre-operative preparation. Psychological preparation vitally important especially for woman of childbearing age anxious to complete family. Sexual relations not impaired by simple vulvectomy.

Skin preparation important. Careful cleansing of vulva with adequate drying and application of antiseptic. Careful shave. Final preparation of skin done in theatre.

Post-operative care. Position. Patient nursed in position causing least tension of suture lines. Low sitting or reclining position with knees raised. Divided adjustable bed ideal. When turned onto side, pillow between thighs and at back.

Skin grafting usually performed after 48 hours with skin taken in readiness from thighs at time of vulvectomy. Following grafting patient lies flat for 72 hours. First dressing done by plastic surgeon often under light anaesthesia. Thereafter area left exposed.

Drain tubes. Subcutaneous drain tubes prevent collection of serous ooze which may be copious for 48 hours. Tubes removed as soon as ooze stops.

Catheter. Catheter in situ allowing free bladder drainage for 3 days then intermittent release of clamp 6 hourly to prevent atony. Catheter removed if bladder emptying satisfactorily on 4th day.

Analgesia and sedation. Used liberally to prevent restlessness and pain for 72 hours. Also allow more efficient deep breathing, coughing, and leg exercises.

Fluids. Intravenous fluids maintained until danger of nausea and vomiting is over then liberal oral fluids encouraged.

Diet. No special restrictions. High fibre diet encouraged to ensure soft, bulky, easily passed motions.

Ambulation. Seventy-two hours after skin grafting patient should be encouraged to move about as freely as possible within her room.

Sutures. No hurry to get all sutures out. Sutures removed as healing becomes quite firm. May be 3 weeks before final ones removed.

Physiotherapy. Breathing and leg exercises encouraged from start. Once patient can move without danger to graft gradually more vigorous exercises started to ensure good posture and mobility.

Discharge. Usually patient ready for discharge by 6 weeks. Appointments made for follow up at 1 month, 3 months, 6 months and 1 year.

Complications. Haemorrhage. Not severe but danger is to viability of graft. Haematomas expressed or aspirated.

Sepsis. Antibiotic cover is usual. Suture lines swabbed with 70 per cent alcohol and dusted with antibiotic powder.

Mastectomy

Usually under domain of general surgeon but often performed in gynaecological unit. Usually for carcinoma.

Operations. Radical (Halsted). All breast tissue, pectoralis muscles, axillary lymph nodes.

Extented simple (Patey). Pectoralis major preserved.

Simple. Breast tissue only.

Pre-operative care. Psychological. Visit from prosthetic expert to match prosthesis with remaining breast. Silastic moulds fitted into custom made brassiere give good appearance.

X-rays taken to exclude metastases in lungs and bones.

Physiotherapy. Adequate preparation essential pre-operatively if patient is to co-operate fully post-operatively.

Skin preparation. Extensive from opposite axilla to umbilicus and round back to midline. Thigh may be prepared for skin graft.

Post-operative care. Position. Elevated to sitting when conscious with arm supported on pillow.

Physiotherapy. Chest and leg exercises started at once with adequate analgesic cover.

Arm movements gradually increased to prevent stiffening and contracture. By 10 days patient should be able to touch back of head.

Wound. Drain tubes. Smaller subcutaneous tube usually superfluous by 48 hours. Axillary tube dressed separate from rest of wound, shortened daily and removed when drainage ceases.

Main suture lines left undisturbed until 7 to 10 days.

Complications. Necrosis along suture lines. Tension on nerve of Bell causing winging of scapula. Lymphoedema of arm. Limitation of shoulder movements. Recurrence of carcinoma.

Careful follow up to ensure patient copes well with psychological trauma from mastectomy and to detect recurrence early.

Index